BOOKS IN THE SPECIAL EDUCATION SERIES

Art Activities for the Handicapped:
A Guide for Parents and Teachers
Sally M. Atack

Better Learning: How to Help Students of All Ages
Overcome Learning Problems and Learning Disabilities
Rosalie M. Young/Harriet H. Savage

Disabled? Yes. Defeated? No.: Resources for the
Disabled and Their Families, Friends, and Therapists
Kathleen Cruzic

Easy-to-Make Aids for Your Handicapped Child:
A Guide for Parents and Teachers
Don Caston

Gifted Children: A Guide for Parents and Teachers
Virginia Z. Ehrlich

Helping Children with Specific Learning Disabilities:
A Practical Guide for Parents and Teachers
Donald H. Painting

Improving the Personal Health and Daily Life
of the Mentally Handicapped: A Caregiver's Handbook
Victoria Shennan

Negotiating the Special Education Maze:
A Guide for Parents and Teachers
Winifred Anderson/Stephen Chitwood/Deidre Hayden

Reading Is for Everyone: A Guide for Parents
and Teachers of Exceptional Children
Dorothy Jeffree/Margaret Skeffington

Special Children, Special Parents
Albert T. Murphy

Special People: A Brighter Future for Everyone
with Physical, Mental, and Emotional Disabilities
Shirley Cohen

Teaching the Handicapped Child: A Guide for Parents and Teachers
Dorothy M. Jeffree/Roy McConkey/Simon Hewson

Understanding and Managing Overactive Children:
A Guide for Parents and Teachers
Don H. Fontenelle

THE WHEELCHAIR CHILD

How Handicapped Children Can Enjoy Life to Its Fullest

PHILIPPA RUSSELL

with additional material by
Nikki Murdick Craft, Ph.D.,
University of Georgia

A SPECTRUM BOOK

Prentice-Hall, Inc., Englewood Cliffs, New Jersey 07632

Library of Congress in Publication Data

Russell, Philippa.
  The wheelchair child.

  (Special education series)
  "A Spectrum Book."
  Includes index.
  1. Physically handicapped children—Services for—
United States.   2. Handicapped children—Services for—
United States.   3. Wheelchairs.   4. Self-help devices for
the disabled—United States.   5. Physically handicapped
children—Education—United States.   I. Craft, Nikki
Murdick.   II. Title.   III. Series.
HV903.R86   1985   362.4'3'088054   84-16050
ISBN 0-13-956020-3
ISBN 0-13-956012-2 (pbk.)

Originally published by Souvenir Press Ltd., 43 Great Russell St.,
London WC1B 3PA and simultaneously in Canada. Copyright © 1978
by Philippa Russell.

10   9   8   7   6   5   4   3   2   1

ISBN 0-13-956020-3

ISBN 0-13-956012-2 {PBK.}

Editorial/production supervision by Elizabeth Torjussen
Cover design © 1984 by Jeannette Jacobs
Manufacturing buyer: Anne P. Armeny

This book is available at a special discount when ordered in
bulk quantities. Contact Prentice-Hall, Inc., General
Publishing Division, Special Sales, Englewood Cliffs, N.J. 07632.

Prentice-Hall International, Inc., *London*
Prentice-Hall of Australia Pty. Limited, *Sydney*
Prentice-Hall Canada Inc., *Toronto*
Prentice-Hall of India Private Limited, *New Delhi*
Prentice-Hall of Japan, Inc., *Tokyo*
Prentice-Hall of Southeast Asia Pte. Ltd., *Singapore*
Whitehall Books Limited, *Wellington, New Zealand*
Editora Prentice-Hall do Brasil Ltda., *Rio de Janeiro*

Contents

Preface

I have written *The Wheelchair Child* with a view to helping and informing parents and professionals about the problems, possible pleasures, and potentials of a wheelchair life. No one study is definitive. I hope that readers will see the book as being a signpost to services and resources, and that they will above all share my firm conviction that wheelchair children are children first and disabled second. Nobody can minimize the difficulties of living with a permanent disability—but wheelchair children can achieve emotional, educational, social, and vocational successes *if* they have the opportunity. Opportunity may mean positive discrimination. It certainly may mean challenge—and all of us who are parents of a handicapped child understand the difficulties in avoiding overprotection and actually encouraging our child to be independent.

When referring to the child throughout the book, I have generally used the pronoun "he." This is necessarily an arbitrary choice; the masculine gender of course refers to both sexes. I have also in general talked about "the mother" when referring to one parent. Nobody could be more deeply convinced than I am that children need *two* parents—and that handicapped children in particular need a father even more than their able-bodied counterparts. But in our complex industrial society, it is still usually the mother who cares for house and child and who attends hospital, clinics, and other sessions on the child's behalf. When saying "mother," I am of course referring equally to father, grandmother, aunt, uncle, or even housekeeper. I hope that my book emphasizes the need for any handicap to be seen as a family affair, and that it will be useful to all members of the family.

I would also like to thank all the parents who have contacted me through the Voluntary Council for Handicapped Children with information queries about services, rights, and needs of handicapped children. They have taught me that many parents find themselves desperately ill-informed about sources of help for themselves and their children. These inquirers have identified gaps in information that I hope this book will help to rectify. Additionally I have been educated—and frequently humbled—by the courageous and optimistic outlook on life shared by many parents and their wheelchair children. I would like to think that this book may help to expand the horizons of families with a wheelchair child, and that it will in addition help the many professionals who *do* care to care more effectively in the future.

I would also like to express my gratitude to all the friends, colleagues at the Voluntary Council for Handicapped Children and the National Children's Bureau, and the parents' groups who specifically answered *my* queries and who offered so many constructive suggestions about the content of this book.

Finally I would like to thank my own three children, Simon, Christopher, and Emma, for their share in this book—Christopher for his line drawings to illustrate the text; Emma for all the precious Saturdays lost because I spent them working on *The Wheelchair Child*; and Simon and all the other children like him who have to live their lives with a disability.

ACKNOWLEDGMENTS

Grateful acknowledgment is made to the National Children's Bureau and its designer and photographer George Clark; the Handicapped Adventure Playground Association and Camilla Jessel; Queen Elizabeth's Foundation for the Disabled; Braune of Stroud and the Associated Newspapers and the National Star Centre for Disabled Youth for the use of the photographic illustrations in this book.

Grateful acknowledgment also is made for permission to reproduce written material from Pauline Skelly, "An Exercise in Integration," *Integration of Handicapped Children in Society*, edited by James Loring and Graham Burn, Routledge & Kegan Paul in association with the Spastics Society, 1975; Maureen Oswin and *Parents' Voice*, National Society for Mentally Handicapped Children; Elizabeth Newson, "Parents as a Resource in Diagnosis and Assessment," *Early Management of Handicapping Disorders: IRMMH Reviews of*

Research & Practice 19, edited by T. E. Oppé and F. Peter Wood-ford, Associated Scientific Publishers, Amsterdam and Elsevier North-Holland Inc., New York, 1976; Mervyn Fox, "Review: The Special Educational Needs of Physically Handicapped Children," *Child Care, Health & Development*, Vol. 2, No. 1, January-February 1976.

1

Some Causes
of Handicap

Mary Sheridan's definition, adopted by the Sheldon Committee in 1967, describes a handicapped child as "a child suffering from any continuing disability of body, intellect or personality likely to interfere with his normal growth, development and capacity to learn." All handicaps vary in severity, and among the handicapped, wheelchair children usually form a minority group.

Handicaps in childhood fall into four basic categories: *Physical handicaps* affect a child's physical functions and general mobility; *mental handicaps* affect intelligence and the ability to learn new skills; *sensory defects* prevent the child from seeing or hearing normally; and *emotional handicaps* (which distort judgment and personality) can exist in conjunction with a range of other handicaps. Most handicapped children suffer from more than one handicap: Many children with cerebral palsy have partial hearing; children with

1

hydrocephalus frequently have either a mental handicap or visual difficulties. Therefore a child's major handicap must be seen in conjunction with his overall development. Many children appear to do badly at school and appear uncommunicative because it has not been realized that they cannot hear properly. Medical advances have reduced the incidence of some kinds of handicap, and can treat others, such as spina bifida and hydrocephalus. Unfortunately treatment is rarely a total cure, although early detection is important in order to start treatment as soon as possible. Since handicapped children are individuals, like all children, the severity or the degree of handicap is not a guide to future "success" in life. With good treatment, education, and family support, very severely handicapped people have done remarkably well in many and varied fields.

It is however, useful to know the main categories of handicap that result in major mobility problems, and to look at the particular problems presented and how they can be solved. Although there may not be a "cure," parents and family can do a great deal to help the wheelchair child enjoy life and experience challenges and opportunities. Many very severely handicapped people live independent lives from wheelchairs; in the end it is often not the wheelchair but the person inside who is the barrier to a more active and exciting life. Parents and professionals have a great (and sometimes exhausting) responsibility to ensure that the wheelchair child does not "think handicapped," and that they expect enough from him despite his disability.

BRITTLE BONES
(OSTEOGENESIS IMPERFECTA)

Osteogenesis imperfecta is the name of the most usual cause of "brittle bones" and a tendency to fractures in children and young adults. It is inherited, and it is estimated that about 7 in every 100,000 births are affected. The immediate cause of the defect is a fault in the protein structure of the bones. Most babies with the disorder will show signs of fracture at birth, and fractures will continue to occur throughout infancy and in the early years of life. Some children will experience as many as 100 fractures, and these may be caused by such trivial incidents as turning to close a door, moving in bed, or being picked up awkwardly. Many parents describe their children as "china dolls"—they hear a crack, a cry, and the child falls down. The "china doll" appearance is increased by the fragility of

2

the skin (which frequently has a translucent appearance) and by the very blue sclera of the eyes.

The condition usually improves as the child gets older, but he will normally show the characteristic deformities of the condition, caused by the softness of the skull, and the fractures themselves. Limbs are usually shortened and the back humped, so that the child may appear "dwarfed." Although nothing can be done to improve the fundamental bone disorder, surgery is useful for some children. The bones are refractured and set straight, with a metal rod passing through the cavity of the fragments. The rods have to be replaced if the child grows significantly, but they prevent further fractures and make walking a real possibility. Most children are of normal intelligence and may cope very well with the psychological and physical problems of the disorder.

CEREBRAL PALSY

Cerebral palsy is perhaps the largest category of physical handicap in childhood. It directly affects a child's movement because of damage to the part of the brain which controls motion and the tension of the muscles. Damage to these movement mechanisms will mean that the muscles may be very stiff (literally spastic) or very floppy. The cause of cerebral palsy may lie in the prenatal period, if the mother contracted an acute infection such as German measles. Very premature babies are more susceptible to this kind of brain damage than full-term infants, and a few children may have a malformation of the brain itself. Cerebral palsy will not necessarily be obvious at birth, when limb tone varies greatly in different infants. It will be noticed gradually, because the baby remains "floppy" at stages when he should be gaining muscular control, or because he shows abnormal movements. Cerebral palsied babies may also have difficulty in eating, sucking, and in talking because of their inadequate muscles. The degree of the disability will vary greatly, and many children will be minimally affected. Others will be very severely handicapped— some with mental as well as physical disability—and will be virtually confined to a wheelchair for life.

Cerebral palsy falls into three main categories:

Spastic children (who form about 50 percent of all cerebral palsied children) have abnormal and increased muscle tension, which makes movement difficult according to the particular muscles affected. Some children

3

have difficulties with feeding, speaking, and may dribble continuously because they cannot control their saliva or swallow easily. The muscles which draw the arms and legs close to the body are frequently also affected, and because of their contraction the hands may be poorly positioned with bent wrists, so that manipulation is difficult. If the leg muscles are affected, the child may walk forward on his toes, with knees bent and the legs crossing in a weaving or scissor gait.

Ataxic cerebral palsy is due to damage to the nerves which descend from the equilibrium centers of the brain. The child has therefore great difficulty in balancing. Many cerebral palsied children seem ataxic at times, because their poor muscle control makes them appear to move in a jerky and uncontrolled manner. But in true ataxia, the child lacks balance in a variety of situations. He may not be able to judge distances, will fall and trip easily, and will need a good deal of help in adjusting to his environment.

Athetoid cerebral palsy is characterized by constant wriggling and writhing movements which the child cannot control. The child is usually floppy and lacking in movement in the first year of life. Then he begins to show the constant writhing, twisting, and grimacing, which are the physical manifestations of the condition. Despite their sometimes bizarre appearance, many children with athetoid cerebral palsy are of normal or high intelligence. Because the areas of the brain involved are some distance from the parts of the brain concerned with intelligence, they can develop well intellectually if physical solutions are found for their often profound communication problems (many athetoids are additionally deaf or partially hearing). The development of new sophisticated electronic aids have radically improved the educational opportunities available, although a large percentage of the more severely affected children need a good deal of help in everyday living.

There is unfortunately no cure for cerebral palsy, but the minority of children who have become cerebral palsied after birth—usually through injury or infection—may make considerable improvements. The majority of these children will probably have *hemiplegia*, that is to say, they will have one affected side of the body and their physical ability will be unaffected on the other side. Hemiplegic children can often attend normal schools, and their disability may present itself primarily as clumsiness. In *quadriplegia*, all four extremities (arms and legs) are affected. In *diplegia*, the four extremities are also affected, but the arms are less affected than the legs. In each type of cerebral palsy, the degree of neurological handicap depends upon the extent of the damage rather than on the type of cerebral palsy.

Even if there is not a cure, there is treatment. Physical therapy is essential in order to prevent the child's condition from becoming worse. If a cerebral palsy child lies or sits in awkward positions, he may in time develop cumulative deformities. The unbalanced muscular arrangement can pull bones out of alignment and leave major distortions. These distortions or contractures can be prevented by proper exercise of all the joints in the body. Braces and other surgical appliances can be prescribed to ensure that the limbs and bodies are kept in proper alignment. If physical therapy is unsuccessful, there are a number of surgical procedures for fusing bones or for correcting affected muscles in order to enable the child to move and sit more normally.

Because many cerebral palsied children are of normal intelligence, education is crucial. If physical solutions can be found for communication problems (possible for the most severely handicapped through electronic aids), many of these children can develop dramatically.

PARAPLEGIA AND TETRAPLEGIA

A number of children and adolescents will have been severely disabled through accident: Despite changing regulations and attitudes toward safety on the roads, rehabilitation centers are seeing an increasing number of young paraplegics.

Paraplegia is usually caused by a spinal injury. If the spinal cord is injured below the neck, messages for movement and feeling from the brain cannot be transmitted to the limbs. The person is therefore paralyzed to a greater or lesser degree. *Tetraplegia* is much more serious, since the damage to the spinal cord is higher up at the neck level and all four limbs and possibly the lungs are affected. Tetraplegia is also known as *quadriplegia*, and it is very unlikely that the sufferer will be able to walk.

Spinal injury of any kind requires very specific treatment and attention. Bladder and bowel control will initially be lost, and help will be needed to reestablish a degree of control. If this is quite impossible, various techniques of coping with incontinence will have to be tried out. Because of the paralysis, spinal injury children will need constant turning to avoid pressure sores—the nightmare of any paraplegic. Techniques for avoidance of pressure sores through suitable activity carried out regularly throughout the day and the relearning of basic skills such as going to the toilet or dressing in a wheelchair, will probably best be acquired in the first place in a spinal injuries and rehabilitation unit.

Because it is vitally important to restore skills as quickly as possible—standing and even limited walking are sometimes attain-

5

able—children will probably have to be treated in a hospital on adult wards, for rehabilitation is still a specialist matter. This can cause problems, but the company of other patients with similar problems can compensate to a degree.

An acquired disability also puts the parents in quite a different dilemma from that presented by a congenital disability present from birth. A previously active child or young person will suddenly need lifting, intensive care, and assistance with bodily functions which his parents have probably not thought about since he wore diapers. Families often rally round magnificently in the first crisis; but day-to-day management is a very different affair, with a home ill adapted for wheelchair living and a child whose expectations have been ruthlessly and suddenly shattered. Families need not only practical experience of living with this kind of disability (probably in the "mock apartment" in the rehabilitation center), but a good deal of counselling. Emotional difficulties such as those in coping with a fiancé who was expecting an able-bodied wife, or with the parents' own feelings of guilt or despair, maybe as real as practical problems of access to an apartment or car.

FRIEDREICH'S ATAXIA

Friedreich's ataxia is a disease of the central nervous system, which starts in childhood or adolescence. In the early stages, the child will show only a slight unsteadiness in walking. This will be followed by an increasing awkwardness and clumsiness of the hands and difficulties in manipulation. The unsteadiness is progressive, and within a few years the child will probably have to use a wheelchair. Vision and hearing usually remain unaffected, but speech can become indistinct and slurred. Although fine finger control, as in writing or needlework, may become difficult, the condition is not usually progressive to the point of permanent immobilization in bed.

Because the condition is inherited, other children in a family may be affected, and early symptoms of clumsiess or unsteadiness should be watched for. Many children will show heart abnormalities, and there is a higher incidence of diabetes in these children than in the normal population. There is no known treatment, but physical therapy can play a useful (if limited) part in maintaining mobility and helping with adjustments to everyday living.

HEMOPHILIA

Hemophilia is a relatively rare condition; only about 1 person in every 25,000 will be affected by severe hemophilia. The condition is a disorder of the normal clotting mechanism of the blood, genetically transmitted through both sexes but commonly affecting only men. There are thirteen clotting factors present in normal blood (factors I-XIII), and the deficient factor in classic hemophilia is factor VIII.

Many children affected by hemophilia will never need a wheelchair: Their lives will be relatively little affected, provided that they avoid injury (which can cause joints to bleed internally) and they receive proper treatment. There are a number of hemophilia centers situated throughout the country, which offer special medical, dental, and orthopedic care. Contrary to popular opinion, hemophiliacs do not die dramatically in a welter of blood after scratching or cutting a finger. The problem is to avoid serious damage to muscles and joints by the slow and often insidious internal bleeding which follows knocks and bangs.

The treatment of hemophilia traditionally involved transfusion of "whole" blood to compensate for the internal bleeding and to supply the missing factor and encourage clotting. This treatment was extremely costly and wasteful, since the hemophilic would receive certain components in the blood which he did not need and which could actually be harmful. In 1966, however, it was discovered that liquid plasma could be frozen. When the plasma thawed, a cloudy precipitate called *cryoprecipitate* was obtained. This precipitate is rich in factor VIII and fibrinogen, necessary for normal clotting. Cryoprecipitate injections therefore bring instant relief to most children. They must usually, however, be given in a hemophilia center and can produce antibodies in some recipients. Another major breakthrough was the development of a concentrate of factor VIII, which can be used for home treatment. But the high cost per injection has severely limited the amount currently available.

Severely affected children, however, do not respond quickly to injections of cryoprecipitate of factor VIII. Hemorrhages into muscles and joints are acutely painful and potentially crippling. Knees, elbows, and ankle joints are commonly affected and *hemarthroses* (swelling in the joint or its synovial cavity caused by bleeding) or *hemotomas* (swelling caused by collection of blood vessels) in the muscles are frequent occurrences. In severe hemophilia, these can appear to occur spontaneously, without obvious injury, and require immediate treatment to avoid permanent damage. In many cases the child will have to rest in bed with the limb immobilized. Hemorrhages not only damage muscle tissue, with scarring and contractures, but if large enough, can damage by compression the nerves and blood vessels passing through the muscle. In these extreme cases, the result can be infection and paralysis. Fortunately, modern methods of treatment and quick access to a hemophilia center have eliminated many of the worst aspects of living with hemophilia. But some severely affected children have to spend periods in wheelchairs while their limbs recover or to avoid injury. Although many hemophilic children can attend normal schools, some have to find education where medical and educational needs can be combined. There is, unfortunately, no permanent cure for hemophilia beyond immediate treatment of any hemorrhage by replacement therapy (using cryoprecipitate or factor VIII by injection); immobilization of the affected limb—in bed, and/or in padded plaster of Paris splints or compression bandages; and physical therapy to prevent permanent deformities of the limb. Aspiration of blood from a joint is rarely necessary now, but despite modern methods of treatment some hemophilic children are very handicapped by their condition and need to have instant access to professional care at all times.

MENTAL HANDICAP

The large majority of mentally handicapped children are in no way physically handicapped. But those who are multiply handicapped will usually be brain damaged during or shortly after birth. Brain damage can arise in a number of ways, but is usually directly related to a lack of oxygen due to asphyxia at delivery, an accident, infections such as meningitis, or a severe form of hydrocephalus or cerebral palsy. With the improvement both in obstetric services and in the care of the baby in the neonatal (immediate postbirth) period, most severely mentally and physically handicapped babies are identified early. Unfortunately, there is seldom any dramatic cure, and treatment is largely good management, early education, physical therapy, and family support. Traditionally many of these severely handicapped children have been regarded as "vegetables." Maureen Oswin, writing in the Royal Society for Mentally Handicapped Children and Adult's journal, *Parents' Voice*, said:

Perhaps our attitudes are coloured by fear; we may be afraid when we see a child who cannot speak, cannot hold anything in his hands, cannot walk or feed himself. We may be embarrassed that the human body can be so grossly incapacitated. If we are so afraid and embarrassed that we want to reject these children as "vegetables," then it is usually because we have no understanding of them as *children* and find it difficult to admit that they really are children underneath their handicaps.

Maureen Oswin's point is a very valid one, since the severely and multiply handicapped child is the most helpless and the most isolated of all handicapped children. Yet, precisely because these children cannot communicate, they are at great risk of being misunderstood, understimulated, and even "forgotten" as children. The parents of these children need enormous support; so do the nurses and staff of hospitals and homes where many currently live through childhood into adult life. But children' units have shown that many profoundly handicapped children can be helped to develop at least to their limited potential.

The majority of these children will attend special classes attached to schools for the severely or profoundly handicapped child. Special classes usually offer special treatment facilities—speech therapy (for feeding as well as speech problems), physical therapy, hydrotherapy if there is a pool, and in many cases a functional training program for the acquisition of basic skills such as toilet training, feeding, dressing, and playing. Unfortunately, special classes end at sixteen for many children, unless they are fortunate enough to live in an area where special classes are incorporated into adult training centers for the more able mentally handicapped adults. Most of these children will not become independently mobile, and their use of a wheelchair will be dependent upon an assistant to push it. Powered wheelchairs require a degree of skill to operate them successfully, although some children will manage to use them to a limited extent.

IQ is an emotive phrase for many parents, but the severely physically or mentally handicapped child is likely to present an IQ of around 20 to 40.[1] Many severely mentally handicapped children are additionally partially sighted and hard of hearing (although these

---

[1] Although most parents are anxious about their child's IQ, in the higher ranges it is rarely significant unless considered in conjunction with physical and other abilities. Many physically handicapped children—like their normal counterparts in the community—have IQs at the lower range of what is regarded as normal (about 80-90 upwards). These children are not mentally handicapped, although they are underfunctioning for a variety of reasons.

sensory difficulties may be hard to discover). Their development is therefore further impeded. Severe handicap is, in fact, almost always a cluster of handicaps and not a single major handicap. For this reason, parents need to be careful observers of their own children. The child with major temper tantrums and a known low IQ may be disturbed because of the physical origin of his problem; he may also be almost totally deaf, which will cause enormous frustration in any attempt to communicate. Some mentally handicapped children have serious behavior problems—such as head banging and self-mutilation—which will need advice from a psychiatrist or psychologist. But others may be behaving abnormally because of secondary problems—reactions to drugs given for epilepsy, problems with sight or hearing or simply manipulation! If a child cannot communicate, it is particularly important that the parents keep some sort of record—noting when bad behavior occurs, when interest and excitement are shown, recording when the child makes a new step forward. If progress is very slow, it is often overlooked altogether. A diary helps to avoid this and also provides backup information for the doctor and school. Many schools for the mentally handicapped keep a home and/or school diary, which travels back and forth with the child, to ensure that parents and teachers know what is happening and how they can help one another.

Because severe mental handicap combined with physical handicap is almost certainly the most difficult category of handicap which parents will encounter, it is worth reflecting that the prospect for these children is not as bad as it used to be. New learning techniques for self-help skills like toilet training, speech, and so forth, are constantly being developed. Behavior modification (basically social training to eliminate bad behavior and teach appropriate actions and response) is increasingly being used with good results.

The severely mentally handicapped child will continue to need a lot of support and supervision as he grows up—and he will continue to need care and support in adult life. Those who are multiply handicapped will always have to depend to varying degrees upon help with dressing, toileting, washing, and so forth. Some will need supervision to make sure that they do not have accidents. However, a number will learn to speak (with a limited vocabulary), to respond to people and places and to do simple jobs without supervision. Those with a lesser mental handicap, even with a major physical handicap, will achieve much more, provided that they have the opportunity to learn and to live in a pleasant and stimulating environment. Wheelchair mentally handicapped adults are a minority group; in the past they would normally have died in infancy from uncontrolled epilepsy or from other illnesses. Most areas have local branches of the National Association for Retarded Citizens and all area health authorities now have community mental health centers. Both can act as pressure groups for better services. Parents of mentally handicapped children have to be joiners!

MUSCULAR DYSTROPHY

It has been estimated that in the United States there are several thousand children who suffer from chronic handicapping conditions in which muscular weakness is the major cause of the disability. About half these children are boys with the Duchenne type of muscular dystrophy. Neuromuscular diseases are basically disorders of the central nervous system involving one or more parts of the "motor units." Motor units consist of the motor nerve cells (or neurones), their nerve fibers (or axons), the neuromuscular points of contact between nerve fiber and muscles, and the cells which are the muscle fibers themselves.

There are, in fact, a range of neuromuscular disorders. Muscle weakness is the common denominator, making the muscles very wasted. Sometimes this is not obvious in a very young child because of plumpness. But young children will show symptoms of clumsiness, difficulty in moving or feeding, or a strange walking gait. Duchenne muscular dystrophy is the most frequent and severe form of muscular dystrophy. It will affect only boys (but is transmitted through the female side of the family). Genetic counselling on the birth of further children, and on the children of any sisters of an affected boy, is crucial. But unfortunately many families will have two or even three children by the time the condition is recognized and the diagnosis made. The clues are usually general slowness in walking, coupled with clumsiness in the preschool years. Boys will tend to fall easily and have difficulty with stairs. Ironically the boy may look particularly fit during these early years, since the calf muscles seem unusually large. The enlargement is not, however, due to the muscular sturdiness of "football players' legs," but to useless fatty deposits. As the symptoms grow, the child will begin to walk with his abdomen stuck out and back hollowed. He may pick up his feet carefully and adopt a kind of waddling "duck" walk. Most characteristic of all is the way in which an affected child will get himself up from a fall. He will normally roll onto his stomach, stick his bottom in the air, push with hands and knees, and proceed to "walk" his hands up his legs until he is upright.

Because muscular dystrophy is a degenerative condition, it places enormous emotional strain on the family. However, despite the adults' natural misgiving and anxiety on behalf of the child, it is essential to keep him mobile for as long as possible. The child has to be encouraged to keep walking; to pick himself up; and, where possible, to lead a normal life. Because of the weakened muscles, splints, braces, or surgical corsets to prevent distortion of the back (scoliosis) or the leg muscles may be required.

Appliances may also be needed when the child is in a wheelchair, to support the neck or hold the legs in a suitable position.

The progress of the disease is fairly predictable. By the time a boy is eight or nine, he will be showing marked curvature of the spine and will probably use the "toe" walk. Between eight and eleven, he may have to start using a wheelchair. Hands are usually affected after the legs, but gradual loss of movement will be experienced. Between the ages of sixteen and twenty-five, deterioration may also affect the muscles of the face, hands, and respiration, and the adolescent is very exposed and vulnerable to infections. The strain on the heart is also considerable.

Many families experience tremendous difficulty in coping with such a severely handicapping condition at home. There are, however, a number of excellent special schools, day and residential, which offer a wide range of activities and nursing care. In its final stages, the illness will require twenty-four-hour attention, if only because the patient needs frequent turning in bed, day and night, in order to avoid sores and cramps.

MULTIPLE SCLEROSIS

Multiple sclerosis is a condition which affects older adolescents and adults: It is a disease of the central nervous system, which affects the nerve fibers.

Nerve fibers have an insulating and protective covering, which is called the myelin sheath. With the onset of multiple sclerosis, this sheath can be damaged and even totally destroyed, and the result is rather similar to damage in an electrical circuit: The fibers stop conducting messages, and the muscles therefore cease to function correctly. Multiple sclerosis varies greatly in the degree to which it affects sufferers, however. The usual first symptoms are weakness in the limbs, balance problems, spasms, and cramps. Sometimes there is blurred vision and difficulty in speaking. Depending upon the nerve coverings affected, there may be strange symptoms of coldness or heat, imperfect sensation, and sometimes a degree of incontinence.

However, despite the possible severity of early attacks, multiple sclerosis is not a continuous condition. Most people have remissions when they regain lost function and feel much better. Remissions can last for periods of years, but deterioration through successive relapses can equally be quick and progressive. Precisely because it is impossible to forecast the progress of the condition, multiple sclerosis excites extreme fear in most families. Since there is no obvious explanation for its origins, nor currently any cure, sufferers frequently get very depressed. The onset of the illness is most likely to be noticed at a stage in the life cycle when young people are eagerly anticipating careers, marriage, or homes of their own. Many multiple sclerosis sufferers are in fact able to work and marry, and some have children. But the likelihood of there being gradual deterioration over a period of time will require considerable courage and objectivity in planning for the future.

Although there is currently no cure, some multiple sclerosis sufferers find their health considerably improved by taking regular doses of sunflower oil (available in capsule form) and following fairly rigid diets and rest patterns. Experiments are also taking place in the United States and the United Kingdom into the stimulation of the spinal cord with an electrode implant connected to a pacemaker. The implant is not unfortunately a miracle cure, as it is suitable for only a limited number of patients. But it seems reasonable to hope that future research will produce similar improvements and techniques to facilitate a more normal life. Meanwhile, it is sensible for any young adult with multiple sclerosis to adapt his home as far as possible to meet his needs when the disease is active, in order that he may make the most of the long periods of remission which most sufferers will enjoy. An American study of multiple sclerosis patients over twenty-five years found that at the end of that period two-thirds were still able to walk. The outlook therefore is one of cautious optimism.

POLIOMYELITIS

Polio can be regarded as one of the few "success stories" among the major handicapping conditions affecting the central nervous system. The development of vaccines in the 1960s has ensured that children (in theory at least) can now be totally protected. In the Western world improved hygiene and sanitation have also eliminated most of the potential breeding grounds for the virus. However, with air travel and increased world mobility, it is still possible to be exposed to infection. Present reluctance to undertake vaccination programs because of possible brain damage will increase the likelihood of cases reemerging. The majority of current polio victims suffering from a handicapping degree of paralysis are adolescents and young adults. Poliomyelitis is not a progressive condition, and the major practical problems lie in adjustment to a severe degree of disability.

RHEUMATOID ARTHRITIS
(STILLS DISEASE)

Acute rheumatoid arthiritis (or Stills disease) can affect children as well as adults. Its earliest onset can be as early as two or three years, and the result can be serious damage and handicap. The basis of arthritis is chronic inflammation of the synovial membrane (joint lining) which produces destructive changes within the joint itself. The symptoms are pain, swelling, stiffness, and tenderness. The affected joints become difficult to move. Fortunately, rheumatoid arthritis varies greatly in its outcome, and 50 percent of all sufferers make a reasonably good recovery. Since no complete cure is known, the treatment concentrates on suppressing inflammation and reducing pain. Orthopedic surgery, physical therpy, and various splints and walking devices may help in individual patients.

In children, the condition is particularly acute because of the possible side effects of kidney or eye trouble. Because children have thicker and younger cartilages in their joints, they may respond to drug therapy more effectively than adults. However, the most effective treatment is still steroid drugs. Until recently, large doses of these drugs stunted growth, and it was not uncommon to see seventeen-year-olds no taller than the average eight-year-old. Now, variations in the dosages have combined a high degree of success in treatment with minimal side effects.

Those children whose arthritis is not contained by rest, physical therapy, and drugs may benefit from the same orthopedic procedures which are used with adults. One rheumatism research unit in the United Kingdom has successfully used hip transplants in young children—although traditionally this operation has been used only on middle-aged arthritis sufferers. Stills disease is a problem for children, who may have long periods of hospitalization and absence from home and school. But since the recovery rate is 70 percent (20 percent higher than for adults), treatment is worth persisting with and expert support is vital. The residual deformities, which were common, can now largely be avoided—although about a third of all affected children will be severely disabled and have a major mobility problem.

SPINA BIFIDA

Spina bifida is one of the more common birth defects in the United States. In 1970 spina bifida occurred in about 3 of every 100 live births. Spina bifida is basically a malformation of the neural tube, which forms part of the spinal cord. In its minor forms spina bifida may be "occulta" (hidden, with little or no physical defect); but "Cystica" (cystlike) spina bifida is more serious and is always obvious from birth. In the less serious type, the *meninges* (the silky linings of the spinal cord) bulge and form a *meningocele* (from the Greek word for a bulge of coverings), but the brain and spinal cord itself are usually normal.

Meningocele, then, is a "sac" that protudes through the bifid vertebrae. It is recognized at birth and causes some physical disability. But the spinal cord remains in the canal and the skin and cord are usually normal. The spinal cord and its neighboring nerves are involved and may be exposed or involved in the membrane cover of the cyst. The cyst or lesion is usually in the lower back and varies in its extent. *Myelomeningocele* is much more serious. In this case the neural groove does not close, and raw membrane and sometimes the spinal cord can be seen until closed by surgery. Depending upon the lesion, there will be varying degrees of paralysis and/or incontinence. It is often (though not always) associated with hydrocephalus. *Hydrocephalus* (literally water on the brain) is caused by pressure building up in the ventricles of the brain by impairment of the circulation of the cerebrospinal fluid. It can also occur without spina bifida, treatment being surgical and involving the insertion of a drainage valve or shunt. Failure to treat or control hydrocephalus can have serious consequences for future brain damage and intelligence, and early intervention is vital. Unfortunately valves can become blocked, or foci for infection, and many children will need special treatment for failures in their valves during early childhood.

Paralysis varies according to the site of the defect. If this is high, there will be considerable paralysis, loss of sensation, and incontinence. The child will be, in effect, a paraplegic. Spina bifida children normally attend special clinics and receive special medical advice relevant to their different handicaps. Physical therapy is important to avoid scoliosis (distortion and humping) of the back and to encourage the child, where possible, to use crutches or propel a wheelchair. Surgery may be involved to correct leg or back deformities. Depending on the degree of paralysis, there are special problems due to the loss of sensation. A child paralyzed from the waist down may easily fall and fracture a limb, lean against a radiator and burn his skin, or simply suffer from pressure sores. Where incontinence is a problem, sore skin will be greatly aggravated by wet incontinence pads or diapers, and a regular routine of hygiene and observation is necessary.

Many spina bifida children have problems of incontinence, and may be susceptible to kidney and urinary tract infections. If there is uncontrollable urinary infection or uncontrolled incontinence in a school-age girl, surgical creation of a urinary diversion may be necessary. Wearing a bag for the collection of urine may seem a terrifying prospect to a parent. But, well managed, it is greatly preferable to the management of incontinence through pads and diapers in later childhood. Incontinence (see Chapter 4) is a major social problem with spina bifida, and professional advice should always be sought on appropriate management.

Many spina bifida children have normal intelligence and are even able to attend normal schools where assistance and modification can be provided to meet their toileting needs. Some of the most severely handicapped have a secondary mental handicap and present considerable problems for their families. If epilepsy, visual problems, and general fragility compound a mental and physical handicap, parents need a great deal of consistent and sensitive support. Studies have shown that there is a higher divorce rate among parents of children with spina bifida, and a very real risk of emotional problems in brothers and sisters.

THALIDOMIDE

Thalidomide was first manufactured in 1954 and was extensively used from 1956 because of its safety as a sedative drug. Thalidomide was ironically unusually safe to the user in the same sense that ten to fifteen times the usual dose could be swallowed with impunity, the patient waking up fit and well the next morning. Because of this apparent reliability, thalidomide was prescribed for a number of pregnant women, and the first "thalidomide child" was born in Germany in 1958. The absence of limbs (known as *amelia*) was ascribed to a congenital abnormality. Other cases occurred, and a special meeting was held in 1961 in Munster to discuss the problems of amelia. Thirty-four children were noted with these limb deficiencies, and for the first time a Doctor Lenz of Hamburg suggested that there could be a connection between the birth of these handicapped infants and the drugs taken in pregnancy, the common factor among which was thalidomide. A similar study was underway in Liverpool, where a Professor Smithells had also noticed five cases of amelia in one year. He checked his records and found that all the mothers had taken thalidomide.

Thalidomide was instantly withdrawn from the German and British markets. The drug company contacted all doctors to warn them of the risks. However, some mothers had of course already taken the drug and had to wait for another six months to see what the results would be. In the end, about 800 children were affected in England, and nearly 2,800 in West Germany.

Thalidomide was destructive to the unborn baby only if taken between the fifth and seventh weeks of pregnancy. It did not affect intelligence, but one dose seemed capable of producing deformities. The results are well-known. The children in most cases failed to develop the long bones of the arms and legs, so that hands and feet were close to the body, giving the impression of "flippers" rather than normal limbs. Many children had malformations of the ears, and some had abnormal heart, kidneys, gall ballader, and other organs. Although a few thalidomide children had fairly minor handicaps, many were very seriously handicapped, and their families had to reorient their lives in order to ensure their progress and the survival of the family itself under the burden. Since thalidomide children, unlike the majority of handicapped children, can attribute their handicap directly to the drug company who distributed the drug, they have received substantial financial compensation—which will be essential for the more handicapped if they are to be helped to function in the community.

Although thalidomide is mercifully a minority cause of handicap, it has alerted both the public and the drug industry to the dangers of any medication in pregnancy; so that a disaster on the same scale is unlikely to happen again. But some children will continue to be born with abnormal development of their limbs for a number of reasons, and the thalidomide tragedy has focused attention upon the problem of children with other forms of *amelia* or *dysmelia* (the technical terms for abnormalities resulting in the absence or shortening of a limb). Because congenital defects of this kind are comparatively rare, it is unlikely that a good service for the artificial limbs and appliances needed can be obtained outside a specialist center. Ideally children will need to make periodic visits to special centers where the consultant, therapist, and parents can jointly determine overall management. Wheelchair chidren with limb deficiencies are normally affected in the lower limbs and may be able to crawl or move themselves around by a shuffling movement (sometimes in a fitting rather like a flowerpot, which can be rocked and rotated from side to side). Other children are able to wear artificial limbs for part or all of the time: Some artificial limbs are now powered and have much greater movement potential than earlier models. However, as the child grows the limbs require careful fitting and constant adjustments to ensure maximum efficiency. Many of the severely affected children have to use a wheelchair for part of the time, particularly for outside mobility. Surgical intervention has improved in recent years, and some thalidomide children have shown how feet can be developed to take over some of the functions of the hands; but the question of whether to operate to achieve one skill at the expense of another may need careful judgment.

2

Help from Hospital and Community Services

BEGINNING WITH A HANDICAP

It has been estimated that about one in fifty babies are born with an obvious abnormality. Some of these defects, such as spina bifida, are serious enough in most cases to involve the immediate removal of the baby to a specialist unit for treatment. Others do not involve immediate treatment, but they need early discussion of a plan for future action with the parents.

There is probably no single area of handicap that excites more criticism, anxiety, and blame than this initial conveying of the diagnosis. Parents in our consumer-oriented society do not expect to have a handicapped child: They assume that the best of medical services will produce the perfect product, the attractive healthy baby seen in the media. The sense of having produced less than this will immediately cause anguish, guilt, disappointment, and a range of feeling difficult to control in the emotional tension of the postnatal period. However, even if parents cannot anticipate a handicap, hospitals can. They have the statistical evidence to estimate the number of damaged children likely to be born in the maternity ward in one year. And while this knowledge may not help the children (beyond ensuring that they are routinely examined, treated, and observed by the appropriate specialist), it can help the parents. One problem is that many hospital staff have difficulty themselves in coping with the disappointment of a handicapped birth, they themselves need counselling and support in order to counsel and support the parents, and when this professional backup is not there, it is hardly surprising that many mothers feel totally isolated and unsupported. Nor is it surprising that they frequently leave the hospital with no clear guidelines for the future. A handicap is a family affair, and unless the hospital has ensured that a source of support and advice is available in the community, a handicap frequently becomes half a family affair, with one or the other parent leaving or opting out.

Part of the problem is the current lack of guidance for a procedure to be followed right from the start. As the English *Court Report* says, "We are in no doubt that parents are entitled to a full and sympathetically given description of any abnormalities or deviations from the normal which have been discovered in their child, and that this should be given as soon as the diagnosis is certain." This task of informing the parents should certainly not, however, be handed, by default, to the most junior doctor or midwife: It should be the clear responsibility of the pediatrician, or of whichever member of staff is felt to be best capable of breaking the news. A plan known as Parent to Parent, for instance, by which the parents of a diagnosed handicapped child are visited by another parent within forty-eight hours of birth, is an encouraging one. The parent is then given the chance to talk to a parent who has experienced this disaster and *survived.* For reality often can prove a great deal better than the future predicted: Parents are still told that the child will be profoundly handicapped, will never talk, walk, work, yet it is rare that a prognosis at birth can be so clear-cut. The importance of this plan is that it offers immediate information and sympathy, combined with a plan for action; it involves the concept that the future still lies in some part in the parents' own hands. They will leave the hospital with information material and invitations to parents' discussion groups. They will also be able to take their child to a special development class, where a physical therapist will ensure that he is handled and stimulated properly. The family is thus "fed in" to the services which can help, instead of being left feeling abandoned in a maze of confusing advice and elusive facilities.

A heavy burden of care undoubtedly falls upon the health and social services in meeting the needs of a family with a handicapped child; but, as the aforementioned plan has illustrated, improvements in services need not necessarily involve a major commitment to new buildings and additional paid staff. The importance of a good service lies in its availability and its capacity to adapt to personal needs. These factors largely depend upon the team work in a particular district and the willingness of the obstetric and pediatric services to cooperate.

Unfortunately, despite a growing professional recognition of their value as partners in the enterprise of caring for handicapped children, many parents are still isolated from the information on which professional decisions about treatment and management are based. As the English *Court Report* notes, they "frequently feel excluded from the treatment régime, caretakers of the child rather than partakers in his treatment." If parents are not sufficiently involved in decision making, they will see the work of the physical therapist, speech therapist, and other professionals as being substitutes for their own inferior care, rather than as means for supplementing and extending this care. Many parents in any case feel timid and ineffectual when confronted by medical practitioners: Traditionally their own families have seen doctors, medicine, and hospitals as special privileged, and omniscient providers of cures. Yet, unfortunately, there is no cure for the majority of handicaps—a confusion for those doctors who see their role as being a curing rather than a caring one; for those parents who cannot accept in their heart of hearts that there *is* no cure. The more handicapped the child, the more they seek a magic solution in therapy. It is not uncommon to meet families whose children have visited every major children's hospital, tried an extraordinary variety of therapies, only to confront disappointment again and again. If they had been better supported at home to put their energies into adaptation and training rather than "cure," would they have searched so hard and so wastefully?

ASSESSMENT

Assessment is an emotive word to most parents—and to many professionals. Assessment will normally begin with the establishment of a clinical diagnosis; that is to say, tests and examinations will confirm

21

that the child has hemophilia, cerebral palsy, or spina bifida. This clinical diagnosis offers basic guidelines for treatment and management. It will not, unfortunately, lead to a particular form of treatment which will bring success or guaranteed improvement. Certain handicaps such as diabetes, epilepsy, or cystic fibrosis can be treated, and often greatly improved, by regular medication. But they cannot be "cured," and the handicapped child therefore presents a particular challenge to the medical profession, who are trained to cure and do not often have the experience and education relevant to the management of a lifelong handicap.

The knowledge that a child has "hemiplegia" or "severe hemophilia" is thus an indicator to certain kinds of treatment and patterns of management, but the importance of the diagnosis will lie not in the "label" tied to the child, but in the functional ability which he can attain. A paraplegic child with no use of his legs, but with strong hand and arm muscles, may be less handicapped in everyday life than a cerebral palsied child with limited mobility but little effective use of hands and fingers. And precisely because it is so important to link diagnosis of a handicap to treatment which is relevant to what residual ability the child still possesses, many areas have special assessment centers. These centers, like the adult rehabilitation centers, look toward rehabilitation and self-sufficiency to the child's maximum ability, and because they are looking at overall development, the physical therapist, speech therapist, psychologist, and audiologist may perform a significant part in the assessment procedure.

The important factors in assessment are *fine motor function* (the use of fingers, coordination of eye and finger movements, and so forth), *gross motor function* (the major physical activities such as crawling, walking, rolling, sitting up, and so forth), *sight and hearing, perception and thought, emotional and social relationships,* and the overall attitude of the child. These skills vary in development in a normal child. In a handicapped child, certain skills may never develop because there is a physical obstacle or a lack of motivation. The child will therefore acquire a secondary handicap and fail to develop to his full potential.

Many studies have clearly shown that a child who is handicapped tends to have other "hidden handicaps" secondary to his major disability. If a child is in a wheelchair *and* short sighted, he will miss opportunities for observation and learning. He may be apathetic because there is nothing exciting to encourage him to be interested. But if his visual defect is diagnosed and treated with glasses, the same child may improve dramatically. Other children are slightly deaf.

22

They do not, therefore, pick up language and may appear retarded and dull. Hearing aids and assistance with lip reading or signing produce marked improvements. The good assessment center will look for these secondary problems and ensure that they are promptly treated.

Assessment is also dependent upon the skill of the parents as observers of their own child. The case history is the foundation of medical procedure, and it is doubtful whether any assessment clinic could provide a complete profile on a child without use of the parents' knowledge of that child's day-to-day living. Everyday skills are important: the ability to hold a cup and eating utensils, to dress and undress, and to get to the toilet unaided. Since the ultimate purpose of assessment is to enable the handicapped person to utilize ability, assessment should also include the family. The majority of severely handicapped people of all ages are cared for at home, so the family's social and emotional problems, be they problems of physical access for a wheelchair, marital conflict, or inadequate income, become relevant to the assessment. The family will also bear the brunt of any recommendations for medical care and treatment.

When a child has been assessed, certain conclusions about his handicap and future development and management will be reached. Unfortunately, many parents feel at this stage that they have gone through a tense and frightening battery of experts who have left them with little to hang onto at the end. If the handicap is chronic, both doctor and patient will have been confronted in the first place with the doctor's limitations: the parents' expectations that a specialist consultant can offer specialist and optimistic advice—expectations based on a misconception that a long-term and chronic condition can be treated in the same way as a short-term and specific one—will have been disappointed. Then, since work for the handicapped is now seen as a collaborative effort, the parents will have encountered a bewildering range of professionals. Expecting reassurance from the fact that their child is under the care of a consultant, they may not understand why the consultant appears to have delegated his responsibilities to the physical therapist, for instance.

So parents need at this stage to be clearly and concisely told what the diagnosis and individualized plan for their child is and what roles the various specialists can play. Only then can they understand their own role in helping their child.

Many consultants now hold a case conference after the assessment. The parents attend and are free to ask questions and discuss any issues. Then, because most people have problems about recalling issues discussed at a time of great distress, the parents also may get a second chance to discuss the assessment's conclusions with one of the therapists or social workers who are present. Second chances are important for parents. If they have not fully understood their child's handicap, they may be open to the varied and frequently wild suggestions of their neighbors and friends about treating their child. And they may not appreciate how crucial the treatment of the child is in the home—how important to avoid harmful positioning and to establish proper feeding, sleeping, and sitting routines, so that they become habitual and thus a form of ongoing treatment.

Because we have in the past been conditioned to *hospital* treatment for a handicap, many parents find it difficult to accept the extent to which they themselves can help their child. They feel safer handing their child over to a professional, so the follow-up appointment after assessment is another opportunity to stress again that it is the day-to-day management of the child that will be his most important treatment. This appointment should ensure that the parents do know how to handle their child, that they understand what is wrong and why the child has the physical disabilities so diagnosed, that they can use this knowledge to help their child, and that they can have continuing contact with *somebody* to discuss developments, problems, and any details of everyday living which are problematic.

Perhaps the key to the problem is mutual respect and communication. If parents feel that they tend to be left in ignorance because they are tongue-tied when in the presence of professionals, the answer may be to *write questions down* before each appointment. Some parents keep diaries, in which they note problems and questions. Many of these problems will resolve themselves or turn out to be ordinary problems of child rearing. Others will persist. Difficulties with positioning for feeding, bathing, or playing may need help—and often a five-minute demonstration will reveal the problem, and a solution. But it is important that no parent leaves an assessment clinic or follow-up appointment unsatisfied. As recommended, assessment must be followed by both ongoing review and advice on management. If these do not follow, the parents' hopes have been falsely stimulated. They have had a problem confirmed, without any assistance to adjust to it or to seek a solution.

Parents may argue that in their area, there are no proper facilities for assessment or review. Their child may have to travel hundreds of miles to specialist clinics to receive treatment (particular for orthopedic deformities or spina bifida). Unfortunately, some children with minority handicaps will have to use specialist facilities, and this will mean traveling and inconvenience for the family. On the other hand, *all* handicapped children can use local services for routine needs such as health reviews, aids and appliances, and physical therapy, and these services should be flexible enough to meet individual needs.

An example of what a good service can mean, when assessment and support are directly linked, is *Honeylands*, a family support unit in England. Honeylands is part of a district general hospital, but it is unusual in offering parents an integrated service of assessment, treatment, and short-term care for handicapped children. Basic to the work of the unit is the belief that each specific handicap or functional disability in a child requires an individual approach which is best started at home. The unit accordingly has "developmental therapists," who work with parents in the children's own home. The therapist will thus be in a position to encourage the family to find its own best way of coping with a handicapped child. At the same time, the wide resources of the unit are available for those parents who wish to bring their children in for therapy and to make contact with other parents. The majority of children attend by day; a few are weekly boarders. But the basis of the service is a common philosophy of care initiated by the staff of the unit, implemented both by parents and themselves, and reviewed regularly and informally. Medical clinics for review of progress are regularly held and are attended by the pediatrician, ophthamologist, specialist in audiology and speech, and so forth. The idea of a sensitive and flexible team is not new in theory but in practice it is rare, and Honeylands offers one example of the kind of service that most parents would like to have access to, if they could. It is highly personal, it is continuous throughout childhood, and it is flexible. Most importantly, it recognizes the need for a handicap to be treated, not in a traditional acute hospital setting, but as a community affair in which the professionals and parents can perceive one another as partners rather than as professional and client.

TREATMENT AND CARE

The General Practitioner

The general practitioner is the cornerstone of health care for the majority of families. Unfortunately, his or her knowledge of the implications of any individual handicap is likely to be as limited as that of the parents when they gave birth to a handicapped child, for the doctor will find it extremely difficult to justify the time and effort spent in gaining knowledge and experience in the management of a handicap that may be encountered only once or twice in a professional lifetime. In a group practice, it is possible that one partner may have a special interest in handicapping conditions. But in a single-person practice, both doctor and patient will become much more aware of their limitations when dealing with a handicap. Because of his limited experience, a general practitioner may thus be reluctant to intervene if a child with a valve for hydrocephalus runs a high temperature. He may argue to himself that a blockage of the shunt could account for abnormal symptoms and prefer to refer the child to the local hospital. The parents, on the other hand, may feel resentful and annoyed that they are committed once again to a trip to the emergency room, where they may in turn be made to feel that their own doctor should be dealing with the case.

In normal acute illness, the doctor can often act out his expected role. He can prescribe medication and act decisively. But with a handicap, nothing will make the problem go away. The general practitioner's role will therefore be more complex, concerned with helping both the child and the parent in a way that lies outside normal practice. He will have to learn to switch from specific medical advice to advice on general everyday living—which is what most concerns the family of a handicapped child. Additionally, a handicap is time consuming; parents will need a lot of the doctor's time not necessarily at times most convenient for the doctor. Because this time is seldom available in a busy practice, doctor and parent may often part with feelings of irritation and dissatisfaction. For just as doctors are not taught how to talk to ordinary people, the patients are often very bad at talking to doctors.

There is no immediate solution to the problem, beyond the hope that parents and doctor will work at their relationship. On the whole parents will have to accept that the special medical needs of a handicapped child must be met at the general hospital.

Therapy

Although doctors are concerned with diagnosis and treatment, much of the actual curative work for handicapped children is carried out by therapists. *Physical therapists* are specially trained to carry out physical treatment to help remedy the physical aspects of illnesses and injuries. Treatment methods vary according to the particular problem. *Passive* treatment involves palliative or supportive measures to ensure that paralyzed or malfunctioning limbs do not deteriorate. The mother or child will be taught how to massage and manipulate limbs in order to avoid the development of deformities and to avoid stiffening of joints. In *active* treatment, a variety of techniques including hydrotherapy, massage, manipulation, and therapeutic movement are utilized to work through a rehabilitation program with a child. The first objective is to identify functional ability and develop this ability to its maximum potential. Second, the physical therapist is skilled in physical assessment and will observe and comment upon development and needs. Physical therapists are also closely involved in decisions about aids and appliances, crutches, and artificial limbs; and in managing the day-to-day skills of feeding, dressing, and bathing.

Physical therapists are increasingly employed as part of the school health service. By going into the school, they can more effectively observe the child's movement patterns within an educational setting and help and assist the teacher. Many parents, however, still complain that information does not filter back to them, unless the child is capable of providing a commentary. It is hoped that area handicap teams will in the future offer a better opportunity to parents to discuss their child's treatment and relate to the home scene. Physical therapists are important to parents, not only for what they can teach the child, but for what they can demonstrate to the parents in the way of lifting and handling handicapped children.

By assessing the home environment against the child's abilities and limitations, they can also provide invaluable advice on everyday living. In some parts of the country, physical therapists do go into the home as well as playgroups and preschools. Because part of their work is in groups, their caseloads can be larger than would be feasible in the typical hospital clinic. Their work is geared to the practicalities of the child's home environment and to teaching the parents how to work with their children. Physical therapists work with the parents of similar aged children, assess their progress, and encourage the *parents* to experience the success of an exercise and to wish to go on further. Since physical therapists are likely to remain in short supply, many children are not going to receive the service they need unless some kind of collective service of this kind is offered.

Closely associated with physical therapy is the *remedial gymnast.* Remedial gymnasts are usually qualified physical therapists who have proceeded to a further qualification. Remedial gymnastics are therapeutic exercises, linked to recreational or work activities and to rehabilitation. They are normally found in a hospital setting.

There are a number of special forms of physical therapy that have developed along the lines of thought of individual doctors or practitioners. These include the *Peto* method, devised by Professor Peto in Budapest to integrate education and therapy. The Peto method has been successfully used with cerebral palsied children. The therapy uses "conductors" or specially trained teachers who work with groups of children on all-day programs. The children are taught movements in a series of carefully devised rhythms and exercises which are repeated at regular intervals throughout the day. This intensive therapy has been found particularly suitable for some severely and multiply handicapped children.

The *Bobath* method of physical therapy also encourages all-day programs to supplement teaching sessions. This therapy is also frequently used with cerebral palsied children, and a developmental sequence of movement is used with each child. The Bobath Center for Physically Handicapped Children offers specialist training in the Bobath techniques to therapists, and the principles of the therapy are widely used.

Perhaps the most controversial form of therapy is the *Doman–Delacato* method of treatment. This therapy was developed at the Institute for the Achievement of Human Potential in Philadelphia and is based upon the theory that when an area of the brain is damaged or destroyed, the surviving cells of the brain can be trained or "patterned" into taking over the functions of the dead areas. The technique involves intensive and exhaustive exercises by the parents on the child who is "patterned" or moved through a series of movements. Some of these exercises involve the use of a large number of helpers, and their repetition ensures that a major part of the child and parent's day is spent on the therapy.

Few children are cured by any form of physical therapy. The value of the therapy will lie in the restoration of maximum ability to the child and in the prevention of deterioration and any cumulative deformities. Some handicapped children—in particular those suffering from cerebral palsy—may deteriorate without regular therapy because of the spasms and unnatural positions which the handicap imposes on their limbs. Most physical therapists combine a number of techniques and professional ideas in meeting the needs of an individual child, for there is no "cookbook" of techniques that will suit all children, and the success of any therapy largely depends upon the selection of appropriate movements and exercises and the parents' intelligent and sensitive cooperation in implementing a program at home. Nancy Finnie's book *Handling the Cerebral Palsied Child at Home* (Heinemann Medical Books) is particularly useful in indicating basic principles of handling and exercises which are relevant to all handicapped children, not only the cerebral palsied.

Occupational therapists have a rather gentle traditional image suggesting basket-making and stuffed animals. However, their role is changing, and they are now an integral part of any team concerned with services for handicapped children. About 15 percent of occupational therapists work for local authorities, many of them for social services departments. With the increasing number of requests for home adaptations and aids, they are likely to make assessments and report back to the local authority on the need for home improvements and other services. Their therapy is concerned with all aspects of everyday living, at home as well as in the hospital, and they are particularly interested in the use of any residual or minimal skills in self-care employment situations. The occupational therapist can advise on problems varying from the most appropriate knives and forks, to ramps and hydraulic lifts for a wheelchair. Social workers, although their understanding of disability and its needs may be excellent, are not trained to assess functional ability, nor are they experienced in the actual use of an aid.

Speech therapists are vital to a handicapped child's linguistic and social development when there is a speech problem. Speech therapy is concerned with much more than the acquisition of basic speech. Speech therapists can advise on feeding problems and other problems relating to throat muscles—particularly important with many cerebral palsied children. They should be an integral part of any team or clinic investigating a child with a disorder of hearing, speech, or language, since disorders of these abilities are frequently interlinked. When a mental handicap is concerned, they can also assist in the communication of basic concepts and preverbal activities which create a *desire* to talk.

Speech therapists are currently in short supply. Because of this shortage, many children will not receive a full service; however, the specialty is now firmly accepted as one of the most fundamental to the overall development of a handicapped child.

Other Services

The *district nurse* is employed within the community health services to provide home nursing care. This may involve dressings and visits in the postoperative period after discharge from the hospital, or it may involve basic personal care: blanket baths or general assistance in the management of a severely handicapped person at home. However, the basis of the nurse's work will be with the acutely ill, and his or her work with families with handicapped children will probably be principally related to periods of illness and incapacity over and above the normal degree of handicap. In 1974, home nurses attended only 43 cases per 1,000 children under five) a very small percentage of their duties. With the increasing number of forty-eight-hour (or less) discharge after surgery, and with the growing emphasis on home care for handicapped children, there is clearly an unmet need for a home nursing service geared to children. Many parents of handicapped children would welcome practical assistance in the early days with managing an ileal loop or colostomy, for instance, or managing a child in frog plasters, which would come more appropriately from a nurse than from a busy doctor.

Psychiatric services, when necessary, are usually offered on the recommendation of a hospital department. Psychiatrists are qualified doctors who have taken further training in order to become expert in the diagnosis and treatment of psychiatric illness. They are also professionally concerned with mental handicaps, as distinct from mental illness. Usually a mentally handicapped child will see a psychiatrist who is a consultant in mental handicaps. These psychiatrists may hold outpatient sessions in district hospitals (increasingly backed up by community nurses, who visit the homes of families with a mentally handicapped member to give practical on-the-spot advice on management and any difficulties that may arise). Sometimes mental handicap consultants hold their clinics at an institution. As institutions operate on a regional basis and frequently encompass large areas, this may involve travel and time. But if a visit to a specialist hospital ensures that therapists and other professionals with experience in the field of mental handicaps will be available, the time taken will prove useful and constructive.

Psychologists are becoming increasingly involved in the care of mentally handicapped or disturbed children. Psychologists are professionally trained in psychology, that is to say, the study of behavior. A clinical psychologist specializes in the application of psychology to the assessment and treatment of mental illness. Educational psychologists frequently work through schools and are also trained and experienced teachers. The psychologist can often work with parents to understand why a child is behaving in a certain way, and help them to overcome behavior or personality problems. Many psychologists (the following the interest of the research centers in the use of behavior modification and teaching techniques with the mentally handicapped) now work closely with parents and can advise them on practical teaching programs in such problem areas as toilet training, personal behavior, speech, and play.

Child guidance services are provided by the local education authority and the area health authority, through either the school health service or the local hospital service. In hospitals the clinics are usually called *child psychiatric clinics*, and referrals can be from schools, social services, or GPs, as well as from other hospital departments. Many children referred to child guidance services have emotional or learning problems, which may be associated with another disability. They are not "mentally ill" in the sense that parents usually fear, but need special help. This help may well be extended to the rest of the family. For obvious reasons, children's problems are also parents' problems, and the parents will be able to participate in any decisions.

Although the education authority does not usually employ therapists, they are responsible for providing full services and will ensure that these facilities (such as physical therapy and speech therapy) are available. Most of the special school health services (such as physical therapy) are provided in special schools only; the handicapped child at a normal school will probably have to attend as an outpatient at the local hospital. Domiciliary services (in homes or schools) are costly in terms of travel time and professional fees, and few school districts could afford to supply therapists on a one-on-one basis. This means that parents with a child in need of regular therapy which is available at a special school should consider carefully what would be available (and what traveling and absences would be involved) if the child were to move to another neighborhood school on an integrated basis. All schools have certain routine medical examinations, according to state requirements; but routine physical therapy or remedial gymnastics may be available only in the special schools. Some special schools have more frequent clinics for children (or parents) with particular problems, and others serve also as assessment centers, with periodic visits from orthopedists, neurologists, and other medical specialists. Medical facilities vary greatly on a regional basis and according to the nature of the school.

Transport to Hospital, Appointments, and Therapists

Getting to a hospital, waiting there for the appointment, and making the trip home again can be a nightmare problem for parents with a physically handicapped child. Transport to the hospital for appoint-

31

ments with consultants, for physical therapy, and for any special treatment should be arranged by the parent. Some hospital social services departments communicate with voluntary organizations, such as Red Cross, who offer free transport (apart from a nominal charge for gasoline) to and from the hospital. The majority of cars can take a folding wheelchair in the trunk, and the service has the great advantage of flexibility. Some areas have volunteer services, and can find drivers for special visits. These can be located through citizens advice groups or social services.

If transport proves an insoluble problem, complain! As the Handicapped Acts stated, transport should be an integral part of treatment and *must* be provided for patients experiencing travel difficulties in attending hospital and other health services clinics.

Many parents feel that they cannot complain and that the system is immovable. This is fortunately not true. Complaints should initially be made to the local school district. It is sensible to send a copy of this letter, with explanatory details, to the local school district, who will actually handle a complaint and contact the relevant individual themselves, if you wish.

There are in any case wide regional variations in the services provided, but these services will not be improved without pressure to make them a priority. Community health councils also have received complaints about transport from other interested groups—including the large number of elderly people who need frequent trips to the hospital for physical therapy or special treatment—and liaison with other groups can only strengthen the case for action.

Visiting Children in the Hospital

It is now generally accepted that parents are an integral part of any therapy or treatment carried out in the hospital and that they should be there, with their child, for the maximum part of any day. (Ideally, a parent should actually, stay in the hospital, but for many parents of handicapped children—who may need frequent or prolonged spells in hospital—this is impractical.) And it is the agreed policy of the Department of Health and Social Security to encourage parents to visit their children in the hospital without restriction. In 1977 a group of voluntary organizations concerned with the needs of children in and with the special needs of handicapped children, met to launch a national campaign to obtain financial assistance for parents wishing to visit their children in the hospital.

Many parents are surprised to find how expensive hospital visiting can be. Often fares are involved not only for the parent, but for other children in the family. If the distance is great, rental cars, taxis, or train journeys may be involved to varying degrees. An able-bodied child in the community will probably go into the children's ward of the district general hospital for any inpatient treatment. But a child with spina bifida may be referred for treatment. Children with Stills disease (rheumatoid arthritis) or paraplegia may attend special hospitals which provide facilities for half the country. The cost of visiting in these circumstances can be astronomical. As one mother wrote to a medical social worker, "I have reached the stage where I have decided that my child can have no more surgical treatment. I cannot continue to make 100-mile journeys to visit him and to pay baby sitters for the younger children. I equally cannot leave him unvisited in a large hospital ward. Either I must choose to abandon him—or I must abandon the treatment."

Perhaps the major victims of this situation are the low wage earners. Families receiving supplementary benefits can be helped through the Social Security Office, providing that the family's income is less *after visiting* than it was before. The basis of payment is the cost of public transport, unless the circumstances are quite exceptional. Assistance is usually based upon a maximum of one visit a day. If more frequent visiting is required, a written recommendation from a doctor or social worker may help.

Although families with a full-time wage earner are normally exempt from this assistance, the Social Security Office has the discretion to help families to make an emergency journey if a close relative is seriously ill. This help will not be given over a period of time, but can be utilized if, for example, a child is seriously ill after surgery. If the journey is considerable and the income low, it is worth persisting.

If parents are wage-earning, but desperately worried about the financial implications of visiting, they should discuss their problems with their local social services department or the medical social worker at the hospital if there is one. If they are members of a voluntary organization, they may receive advice from them. But voluntary organizations are also feeling the impact of hard times. Besieged with requests for assistance, their resources are stretched and they are unlikely to be able to offer long-term assistance. However, many hospitals have endowment or other private funds which they can use to help with travel and visiting expenses. Application is

33

made through the hospital (usually through the social worker), and the outcome depends upon the circumstances of the applicant and the money available at the time. There are a wide range of small charities throughout the country, which can sometimes give financial assistance to families meeting the terms of their bequests. Some Rotary, Lions, working men's, or other clubs give assistance in case of special need. The Armed Forces have a number of discretionary funds for assisting members' children.

If a child is in a long-stay ward and receiving education in the hospital school, it is possible to get financial assistance from the *education* authority. Under prior regulations, education authorities are instructed to assist parents with visiting if the child's education would otherwise suffer. It is clearly difficult to quantify the educational implications of a parent's failure to visit, but many hospital teachers and social workers are willing to give appropriate evidence and support for an application for assistance. A strong indication of family stress, the difficulties of visiting, and a sympathetic social worker may produce assistance.

Hospital visiting is probably not an issue that many parents consider until they are personally faced with the problem. When they are, they should ask, complain, and campaign to change the current anomalies.

Social Services

Social workers and social services departments offer a major resource to families with handicapped children. Sometimes, however, because of the large share of responsibility for the care of the handicapped which is assigned to them, their resources in personnel, time, and money may be outstripped by demand. Social work is also in general a "generic" (that is to say, general) discipline, so many workers have little practical experience of working with handicapped families—like general practitioners, the majority of their clients are able-bodied. But social workers can, for instance, be expected to give advice on child management (as well as in the provision of aids, adaptations, and financial assistance) and to have extensive contact with local voluntary and statutory services.

Many families gain a good deal of support from social workers. Their training enables them to understand family problems and to counsel and support. They can provide very practical help around the home in the way of aids and adaptations, and perhaps they can provide contacts with local voluntary organizations and preschool facilities, and sometimes financial assistance with hospital visiting or holidays. Some departments run groups or clubs for parents of handicapped children and encourage the parents to adopt a more confident and self-supporting attitude to their child's disability. Although social workers have not usually practiced as specialists, some have become specialists rather than generalists because of their attachment to hospital departments or special schools. In this situation, they are able to acquire a very specialized knowledge of parents' problems and needs and to keep in close touch with relevant facilities in the community.

Parents are often confused about the social worker's role. Some feel that social workers are only for the feckless and incompetent, others that they can't do anything very much to help. It is a reflection of the chronic understaffing of social services departments that few social workers can visit regularly. Their arrival tends to represent a family crisis, and in this emergency situation it is often difficult to arrive at an immediate decision which is acceptable to the family and to the available resources. Ideally, work with the handicapped should be a continuous, and a collaborative effort, so that social workers need to cooperate with doctors and teachers.

It is inefficient and exhausting for parents to have to continually search for appliances and counselling help, together with ongoing medical treatment from as many as five or six different agencies. And social workers, having an ongoing and community-based interest in the families, are perhaps the most likely people to act as coordinators to family services and problems. But in practice, they may find this very difficult.

Unfortunately, parents sometimes see the inability of their social worker to provide all that they require as being indicative of personal inability, rather than of problems with official services in the areas. Many parents move to what they see as a "good" local authority, or sacrifice career opportunities or personal choice to remaining where services are good. If local services appear inadequate, parents themselves can do something to improve them by working together in groups to present statements to social services committees; by making representations—perhaps with regular evening or daytime meetings with the department—about services to be developed; and by informally keeping social workers informed of local voluntary activities and families' needs. Parents' groups are a very economical way of utilizing expensive professional services, and most social services departments are very willing to be involved.

Handicapped children have needs like other children, and it is crucial that they should live with their own families if at all possible. But if parents feel so exhausted that they really cannot cope—what then? Parents are only human, and if they see the point arriving at which they cannot cope, there is nothing to be ashamed about. Social services departments can usually arrange short-term respite care, which can be in an institution or in a hospital. Most handicapped children gain from an occasional break, and it is obviously important that parents should not drain their emotional and physical energies so much that their child eventually has to live away from home for good. Some parents feel very ashamed that their child is going away from home; they feel they have failed, and this feeling is particularly strong if friends or neighbors are tactless enough to imply that they have "put the child away." But if parting, temporary or permanent, becomes a realistic choice (and many teenagers do choose to live away from home, whether handicapped or able-bodied), parents should be courageous and discuss local possibilities with their social services and housing departments. Social workers rely on parents to ask them to meet their needs, and parents have to learn to be frank and courageous in explaining what they want.

If a family can no longer care for a child at home, local authorities may care for the child in special facilities, in integrated community homes, or sometimes through foster parents. Residential care on a long-term basis in a hospital is becoming less common and will usually be approved only if a child has major medical needs. A child will usually stay in a children's home until he is sixteen. He will then move back into the community or into an adapted apartment or an adult group home. Since wheelchair children are such a minority group, it may however be difficult to fit them into children's homes which were adapted from older houses and designed for mobile children: So there are children who live in the hospital who could perfectly and easily be in the community if the access problems could be overcome.

Voluntary Organizations

Voluntary organizations provide a major role in serving the information and practical needs of handicapped people in the United States. A list of useful organizations is given in Appendix A in the back of the book. Voluntary organizations range in scale from small local groups to national organizations with professional staff, a wide range of training and other programs, exhibitions of aids, information service, and so forth. Some parents hesitate to get in touch with voluntary organization, feeling that they must be staffed by well meaning but potentially embarrassing "do-gooders." While it is in the nature of a voluntary organization that it must rely heavily on local goodwill—and labor given gladly and for no charge—most are very professional in their liaison with statutory services, their knowledge of local provision, their ability to counsel, and (sometimes) to provide financial assistance.

A number of societies run social, sporting, and other recreational activities—often with some financial support from local authorities or area health authorities. A number have preschool playgroups or run parent workshops with the assistance of professional psychologists and teachers. Voluntary groups are largely what their members want them to be—and parents who join can be certain not only of the support and experience of other parents with similar problems, but of taking an active role in obtaining the services they desire for their child. Many voluntary organizations are actively concerned with local policies for the disabled; they have representatives on area health authorities, community health councils, social services committees, and school boards of education. Since the handicapped will always be a minority group compared with the elderly, one-parent families, the homeless, and other groups with urgent demands on national and local resources, it is important that they and their parents are joiners. Voluntary organizations, being independent, can argue, cajole—and experiment with residential, training, and other schemes which may later be taken over by local authorities. It pays to participate—even if only to the extent of sharing in a pool of special equipment or toys, helping with a playschool or holiday program, or just enjoying whatever social activities are available. It pays even more to take a keen interest in the way local services are developing and to remember that the three-year-old handicapped child may one day need wheelchair housing and the five-year-old boy a place at an adult training center. Handicap is for life—and families can fight better together.

3

Growing Up
with a Disability

HANDLING THE YOUNG
HANDICAPPED CHILD

The handicapped child is a child first and a disability second. Yet the mother herself is likely to be in a particularly vulnerable state when handling the young child, especially when—as is true in a high proportion of cases—the handicapped child is a first child. Families today are more mobile than they were in the past, so there are rarely relatives or older friends with experience in child rearing to advise on the normal and abnormal, and the young parents tend to feel they are bringing their child up in isolation, combining instinct with information gleaned from the clinic, the media, and baby books. Because a handicapped child may be slower to respond; have difficulty in moving his head so that he can be encouraged to smile or babble; be harder to feed; perhaps spend long periods in the hospital when his mother may not be able to cuddle him because of postsurgery recovery or plaster casts, she may feel that he is not like other babies. And she may, in her turn, fail to give him the cues that a mother usually gives. A child needs physical warmth and comfort. He needs speech and interest when he is being fed and dressed. Especially if he is limited in movement, he needs stimulus. While, in short, a handicapped child is certainly a special child with special needs, he equally has the needs that all children share. So a mother's best guide may be a babycare manual which deals with normal development and normal family relationships.

Development of any child is a continuous process with enormous individual variations, and few handicapped children will develop in a slow steady spiral. They will progress rapidly in some areas and appear more handicapped in others as a result. Then because of their feelings of natural sympathy for the child's disability, or simply because it is so much easier to do it oneself, parents may fail to encourage the development of basic skills. It may seem unkind to encourage a child to be sociable, for instance, if he is severely cerebral palsied and unlikely to speak intelligibly—but if the child is to learn not to hide behind his disabilities but to maximize his abilities, and as far as possible compensate for his handicap in later life, he must be stimulated early and consistently.

INFORMAL EDUCATION— THE PARENTS' ROLE

Small children learn through imitation of their parents. Cuddling, kissing, singing, bouncing, and tickling are common in all cultures. They excite and please the child; they encourage him to relate to one person. The child will learn to communicate through gesture and noise long before he understands selective speech. Early squeals and laughs are preludes to proper speech, for speech itself will never come unless the child recognizes the values of words as a means of communication and desires to relate to other people. Babies, like adults, respond to admiration and encouragement. The child who spends most of his day lying in a bed or stroller has no incentive to see himself as part of the human race. He will learn that prolonged screaming will bring attention of a kind—but he will not learn that human relationships are based on more subtle interactions. Indeed, a child who spends too much time "resting" is likely out of sheer boredom to adopt the attention-seeking or self-abusive habits which are often observed in long-stay hospitals.* He will tear his clothes, pick at his hands, bang his head against the wall, or rock the cot. Disturbing behavior tends to reinforce itself, since it produces adult intervention. It also becomes pleasurable through habit, and thus self-perpetuating.

Young handicapped children should be with adults. They can be propped up on sofas or settees, or sat in one of the range of special seats which are available. The plastic baby chair with adjustable back, or the hammock-like bouncing cradle chair available from baby stores, enable the baby to see more of the world without distorting his back. Cerebral palsied children who cannot lie or sit comfortably on their backs and control their hands because of spasms or reflex movements, can lie on their stomachs on triangular wedges of foam.

On the other hand, sharing the home environment with the child does not mean that the child should be allowed to dominate all activities. It is an overanxious mother who never leaves her child alone, continually jiggling, tickling, and thrusting new toys under his nose. Children need interest, but they do not need a kaleidoscope of confusing attentions. And despite his primary need for his mother— or his "motherer"—a baby also needs love and care from other members of the family. It is easy to feel that nobody can care for a handicapped child except his mother, but children also need fathers. A man's firm hold is of comfort even to a tiny baby; and the physical bond that is established at that early stage is important both to father and baby. The father, in fact, who is excluded from his child's care, and who has in addition to cope with guilt feelings about having an abnormal baby, may literally opt out. Surveys of families with handicapped children have shown that many fathers have gradually, though unintentionally, found themselves thrust into the sole role of provider, mystifyingly excluded from the emotional life of the home. The less they have cared for the child when young, the more they may feel incompetent to do so when the child is older.

Grandparents too can play a major role in a handicapped child's life. Initially, of course, the grandparents may have deeply ambivalent feelings about the handicapped grandchild: They may have looked forward for years to the arrival of the child, and have formulated their own powerful fantasies about the role they would play, doing with him the sporting and recreational activities they never did with their own children, for intance. The handicapped child thus distorts their own self-image, and they too will need time to adjust. But grandparents do care. They have a vested interest and continuing concern in their grandchildren, and above all they have *time*. But if they are to be closely involved, they need to be considered at the very beginning of the child's life. It is much easier to learn to cope with a urinary device or brace on a very small child than a grown one. Limited speech and gestures will be better understood if they have been shared since birth. Additionally grandparents, like the parents, may feel very dubious of their own abilities to cope if they are not involved early.

The same could be said of neighbors. If neighbors avoid the new baby it is more likely to be due to embarrassment and uncertainty than to genuine dislike or lack of care. Straightforward explanations (with the loan of simple leaflets on, for example, spina bifida) will usually produce straightforward attitudes. Although it is hard to have to give health education lessons to explain one's own child, parents who are willing to be matter-of-fact about a disability and to answer questions in a simple manner will in turn secure friends and interest for that child in later life. Many of the wilder misconceptions about physical handicap (based purely upon observed physical differences) can be quickly dispelled in a few sentences.

It is, in any event, important that any handicapped child should from his earliest days observe informal and friendly social contact between his parents and other people. Handicapped children brought up, as many regrettably are, in extreme isolation in a small family unit, tend to appear gauche and stiff as well as handicapped in later life, because they have never observed natural relationships with outsiders. If handicapped children are to be integrated in a normal way, they will need to have acquired a certain poise with and confidence in other people. They are most likely to be able to do this if they have seen friends and neighbors naturally entertained in their own home.

STARTING TO MOVE

A young physically handicapped child may tend to lie in one position and be reluctant to try others. While all children have a favorite position, children with any disability need to be taught to move themselves and to avoid adding to deformity by lack of exercise. Physical therapists can give practical advice on, for example, holding and turning a child and on correctly placing the head. If a child tends to get into awkward positions, baby bumper pads can be purchased from children's shops. These cloth-covered pads fit around the sleeping end of the bed and protect the head from the bars. If a child finds that limited movement is further restricted by bed clothes, he may be more comfortable under a comforter (which will move easily if it has a nylon or other slippery synthetic cover), or with an orthopedic support for the blankets, to form a tunnel for his legs. Children who cannot get themselves into a sitting position should have firm foam pillows (a range of standard safety pillows are available).

Many severely handicapped young children will also not be able to learn to play spontaneously. Mobiles, musical toys, and other attractive stimuli around the crib will be needed to encourage them to use their hands or try and roll over. And most young handicapped babies will need special encouragement to start moving. Physical therapy can demonstrate exercises to initiate basic movements, like rolling over and crawling. These should then be done regularly but not to the point of exhaustion of the child. Little and often are freqently better than marathon sessions which leave child and parents weary and ill-tempered.

CARRYING AND SUPPORTING
A YOUNG HANDICAPPED CHILD

Many young physically handicapped children have poor head and neck control, which makes it difficult to hold them in a normal face-to-face position for play or feeding, or to carry them round the house. There are a number of commercially produced canvas and cloth baby slings which can be worn across the front of the mother's body. These make it possible to carry the child with one hand supporting his head and one hand free for shopping or other activities. When sitting down, if the mother sits squarely in front of a table, and places a cushion or foam triangle against the table with the baby resting on the cushion and facing her, they can play without risk of the child's head lolling, or his body slipping. With a bigger child, one leg can be put round each side of the mother's waist so that there is no risk of a sudden movement causing him to slip onto the floor. This method of seating is also convenient for feeding or for dressing the top part of the child's body.

SITTING AND PLAYING

If a spastic or paraplegic child wishes to play on the floor, there are a range of triangle seats available. These seats support the child, restraining his body with straps, and enable him to play at floor level. If the mother is playing with the child, she may prefer to sit on the floor and put the child between her legs, with his body and head resting against her body. This can be a useful position when a child is beginning to do puzzles or other games on his own, or to dress himself. If the mother adopts an eye-to-eye contact position, the child will probably fix his attention upon her face to see if she is approving or critical. If she sits behind, she can offer guidance but not dominate the activity.

Very severely handicapped children, particularly the cerebral palsied who may have poor hand control, can have great difficulty in learning to use their hands. Games with toys or household utensils preferably involving a variety of textures, and many of the clapping and acting games of childhood like "patty-cake" help a child to use his hands. Since many perfectly competent children will not make an effort to touch or take while there is somebody there to help them, it may be useful to put the child in a comfortable position on a bean-bag-type chair, or in a triangle seat, with a suitable small table or tray, and let him play with toys alone for a while. Beanbag chairs are very useful, since they can accommodate any member of the family, and can be placed in a variety of positions for sitting or prone activities. However, it is important, with any handicapped child, to make sure that a chair or piece of equipment is not actually increasing his handicap by reinforcing undesirable posture. Both the beanbag chair (which is stuffed with polystyrene pellets) and the various triangle and inflatable chairs can be dangerous if a child is tired and slumps forward. Sometimes a combination of seating arrangements is most satisfactory. Car seats can be useful for some children in the house. The older type of car seat (resembling a short highchair with a tray) is rarely suitable for the more handicapped children, but the new car seats with their wide harnesses can be put inside conventional highchairs to give complete support (care should always be taken when using highchairs to ensure that the child can get himself back into an upright position if he slips). Children who are just beginning to sit up and play may actually prefer to sit inside plastic laundry baskets or cardboard boxes. Both have the advantage of being cheap, unlikely to do any damage if knocked over, and light enough to be easily carried from room to room. A conventional playpen is of little use to a very handicapped child except to confine his toys and protect him from other members of the family.

FEEDING AND DRINKING

Cerebral palsied children in particular frequently have difficulty in learning to drink from a cup and to chew food. Many handicapped children are addicted to their bottle for food *and* comfort. This may be partly because the child has spent long periods in the hospital and there has therefore been inadequate opportunity to wean him and partly because the bottle has been a comfort for him. A mother whose child has reemphasized his need to drink every time she visited him in the hospital may also feel that she must continue using a bottle in order to maintain fluid levels. This reluctance to wean will apply especially to babies who have had real feeding difficulties in the early weeks, so that the battle to encourage sucking continues to loom large in the parents' minds. It is not therefore surprising that weaning is often left to a later date than normal, and that the child is in consequence reluctant to use a cup or chew solid food.

A handicapped child's need for vitamins, proteins, and calories is exactly the same as that of his able-bodied counterpart—with the proviso that a wheelchair child will put on weight more easily so needs to be encouraged toward fresh fruit and cheese rather than ice cream, soda, and cake. Most babies acquire the ability to sip from a spoon in very early infancy, even though their major food intake is through the suck and swallow reflex. But some handicapped children have poor tongue control, which means that their apparent swallowing is really simply permitting liquids to trickle down their throats. Although a child may be able to eat yogurt, custard, or soft fruit purees in this way without choking, he will need to master further skills to eat a normal diet. If a child moves his tongue but cannot move his jaws rhythmically in a chewing motion, he will mash food up but not chew it. Instead of swallowing it, as a normal baby will swallow a chewed-up piece of toast, the child will probably choke when food reaches the back of the throat. And since choking is an unpleasant sensation, he will be even less motivated to eat next time.

Messy feeding is often a major irritant to parents in early childhood. However, it is useless to get angry with a handicapped child who cannot control himself properly. If mealtimes are aggravated by the presence of other members of the family, it may be necessary to feed the child quietly on his own until he has achieved some skill. Stressful mealtimes are powerful disincentives to children, and the combination of family comments and mother's anxiety may result in a tense child who will resist any attempt to feed him. Mealtimes can easily enough become battlefields for normal children; it is worth taking a lot of trouble to see that they do not become antisocial occasions for handicapped children.

A speech therapist is often the best person to advise on developing oral control. He or she can suggest exercises for developing coordination of the tongue. Children with poor tongue control will also have problems in learning to drink from a cup or glass, and they are likely to dribble liquid out of one side of their mouth.

A child will not be in a position to swallow properly unless his head is properly supported. A child with a large hydrocephalic head, for instance, with muscular abnormalities or cerebral palsy, may tend to shoot his head back when eating or drinking. This intensifies the chance of choking and makes chewing virtually impossible. If the child is seated facing the parent who is feeding him, with his head and back supported on a cushion, baby chair, or wedge leaned against a firm surface, he can concentrate on the job in hand. (This position is not suitable for a family meal table, since the child will be distracted and will probably arch his back in an effort to look round and over his shoulder.) His jaw movement can be initiated by the parent. It is possible to manipulate the jaw by hand in order to demonstrate the correct movement, and again speech therapists can usually suggest exercises to help develop a suitable jaw action.

A number of firms manufacture plastic tableware for children. Ekco and Be OK! (Fred Sammons, Inc.) both produce plastic spoon and fork sets. They have the double advantage of having shallow spoon bowls, which are easy to empty in the mouth, and are relatively soft if the child slips or pokes his mouth or face during feeding. J. A. Preston Corporation makes special implements with curved handles. These angled handles are particularly useful for children with a minimum of wrist and elbow movement. They are less suitable when the child is being fed by someone else.

For this, especially if the child is a wriggler and particularly unhappy feeder, some parents may find the *chicco* bottle and spoon combination useful. Fairly liquid food is placed in the bottle and squeezed onto the spoon as required. Since the bottle can be squeezed when the spoon is actually in the child's mouth, there is minimal risk of spillage and mess. And if mealtimes are very protracted, it may also be useful to buy one of the many heated plates. These are normally made of unbreakable plastic and have a hot water compartment to retain heat. Most have rubber suction disc bases to prevent them from being knocked over. A wide range of nonslip mats and suction cups are also available on the open market.

Children's cups are available in every size and shape, so it is best to experiment to find the one most suited to the child. Special melamine cups with cutaway handles, which require little finger control, and spouted cups, which do not spill if knocked over, can be acquired from such companies as Be OK! and J. A. Preston. Some children find straws helpful (although a child with very poor lip and tongue control is unlikely to be able to use them without practice; and combined with lidded drinking cups they make a safe way of having drinks in bed or in a prone position.

As a child gets older he may encounter major difficulty in gaining enough control over the force he exerts when he cuts up his food. The plate moves along the table, or tips and spills. The answer here is a nonslip mat. Latex mesh carpet underlay is cheap and can be cut up into mats—it is also useful for stabilizing toys or toilet articles. Or a special material called *dycem* can be purchased, either as mats or in lengths. Dycem is a gelatinous material which is nonslip on both sides. It can be cut to shape as required.

Older children will also want to use normal eating utensils, but may find metal forks and knives difficult to manipulate. These can often be simply made manageable by slipping the handles into rubber bicycle or tricycle hand grips, which can be purchased cheaply from any cycle shop. Foam rubber too can be twisted round cutlery handles, but it is difficult to wash and dry when soiled.

Nobody with weak hand control, too, can manage food easily on a rimless plate, and the substitution of a deeper bowl will often help considerably.

Eating is a social occasion, as well as a means of refueling the system. It is therefore essential that the handicapped child should be able to eat as efficiently and as aesthetically as possible. Bad table manners are a social embarrassment to *all* children if they are allowed to continue. Since wheelchair children will need every friend they can keep, it is important that their eating habits are acceptable and sufficiently relaxed for them to experience mealtimes as the pleasure they can be.

TOILET TRAINING

If a physically handicapped child is not incontinent because of his handicap, he will need the same toilet training as his normal brothers and sisters—that is, he will need to be motivated, patiently and consistently. He may also need some appliance to make him comfortable and safe when using the toilet.

Toilet training is a difficult subject for most mothers, and more so when the child is handicapped. Some mothers feel that a child with mobility problems (or with a secondary mental handicap) has enough to contend with without yet another training regime. But diapers sooner or later become uncomfortable, spoil the look of normal clothes, and (as the child gets bigger) tend to become soggy and cause diaper rashes. It is therefore better to treat the child as you would any other and start at about eighteen months to two years, unless the child himself indicates that he is willing to try younger. Children with older brothers and sisters are often motivated to be like them and to accept the transition from diapers, through in a few cases, the reverse is true and they enjoy their role as "babies" and the physical attention it brings from the mother.

Few children are trained without an interim period of puddles and worse. Unless they are taken out of diapers, they may not even be aware that they are damp, or that being damp is uncomfortable and better avoided. The physical handicap may also prevent a disabled child from getting himself quickly to his potty or toilet. Since most children take time to "signal" much in advance of the act, this may mean a regular routine of toileting or keeping a suitable potty in the room.

Many children's potties are quite unsuitable for a child with balancing problems because they tip too easily. A number of special pots on the market include those which incorporate the pot in a miniature chair with a strap. These are both stable and comfortable, and they have no sharp "lip" to injure sensitive skin. A small commode that is made of wood with a support bar and contains a built-in potty is very stable and enables the child who tends to fall forward or go into a spasm to hold the bar and maintain a safe position. Other small children may actually feel safest if they use a normal toilet with an appropriate toilet seat and side bars for support. Bars or frames to facilitate independence on the toliet, and trainer seats (from Be OK!, Ekco, or other standard brands of children's equipment) can be fitted over the toilet bowl. Be OK! also manufactures a plastic block designed to enable small children to climb up to adult toilet and sink levels. A physically handicapped child may not be able to use this as a step, but he can use it as a foot rest so that his feet do not dangle.

Since all aids and modifications take time to set up, it is also worth considering some makeshift remedies, especially if handicapped children are to be able to travel away from home, since they will not always be within reach of a modified toilet. An ordinary plastic potty is often quite stable when placed inside a large cardboard box. The child can use the back and sides of the box for support. Larger children, who are heavy enough to tip a box, can hold onto the back of a chair. This position is particularly useful for children who are able to pull themselves into a standing position for adjusting clothes.

Children take varying times to toilet train—generally parents feel at the time that their child is incredibly slow; in retrospect they feel certain that the process was carried out in record time! However irritating it may be to have wet diapers—or wet trousers and wet carpets—it is worth persevering. If a child gets to four and is still often damp, the reason may be nothing to do with his handicap. He may, like any other child, have emotional problems. Starting in a playschool or special class may have disrupted his basic routine. He may be jealous of another child in the family, or he may be getting over the aftermath of a period in the hospital.

Many perfectly healthy children arrive at preschool or kindergarten having an occasional accident, so some leeway should certainly be allowed for the particular practical difficulties which may face a handicapped child. If he has difficulties in communication, he may simply find it very hard to get his needs across in time. This will improve. If he has spina bifida, he may not have warning sensations before emptying his bowels or bladder until it is too late. The handicap may in any case increase the gap between "assisted continence:" when the child will use the pot or toilet if sat on it by his parent, and complete control when he goes himself—or indicates that he wishes to go, if he cannot get to the pot on his own. Once a child is toilet trained, he will be anxious to develop this new skill as a solo effort, and it will be worth discussing with other parents, the physical therapist, and occupational therapist, how they recommend that the problem can be coped with. Sometimes a child becomes more self-sufficient if he is in a wheelchair—since he may be able to use his wheelchair to reach the bathroom and transfer himself directly using pulls or rails. In other cases, this may be very difficult. A number of spina bifida children will spend at least part of each day on braces and crutches—but girls may have additional difficulties if their braces cannot bend. The approach to total independence in toileting will, therefore, be a slow one. Different skills will be mastered at different times and—in some cases—will never be totally mastered. The important thing is to be as relaxed and positive as possible and ensure that the child is as independent as his disability allows.

CLOTHING

Young children are fashion conscious from a very early age. They wish to conform to the style of their own age group and, frequently, wish to wear combinations of garments of which their parents heartily disapprove. Handicapped children have an even greater incentive to look like everyone else. But sometimes the desire for fashion has to be modified by the requirements of the wheelchair life—and parents need to remember in turn that dressing a young child in "nice" clothes reminiscent of their own childhood will not necessarily taste or endear the child to his peer group.

Where to Get Clothes

Ten years ago, dressmakers (or willing grandmothers) were easy to find when special clothing was required. But now that the majority of clothes are mass-produced, it can be very difficult to find clothes for particular needs. As children who wear heavy braces, or who are incontinent, will require more clothing than usual, the problem is compounded by expense.

Some chain-store clothing is quite suitable, with minor alterations, for handicapped children. Because dress fastenings are often difficult of access, however, it may be preferable to buy top and bottom separates for girls: Rear fastening can also be uncomfortable for a wheelchair child, and buttons and zippers can actually cause damage and pressure sores. However, fastenings can be quite easily changed for elastic or velcro strip, and the overall fashion appeal of the garments maintained. Another advantage of buying separates is that many physically handicapped children have atypical sizings, and may require very different fittings in skirts and jackets.

Some parents find physical access to children's departments a major problem. The majority of stores have direct access by an escalator or staircase. However, the larger shops also have service elevators, and a preliminary telephone call to the manager usually produces cooperation. Smaller children's clothes can be purchased by mail order, but it is sad for a child never to have had the opportunity of choosing and rejecting clothes in a shop. Many larger stores also have fitters who can alter and adapt garments. If they are not able to do so themselves, they can offer useful advice on home modifications.

Some mothers would like to make clothes themselves, but may have difficulty in altering patterns. If a mother feels that she needs practical as well as theoretical help, it may be possible to go to evening or daytime adult education classes in needlework or tailoring and learn how to make alterations at home.

Since quantity, as well as quality, is often a problem, many parents buy clothes at flea markets and garage sales. For a child who is spending months at a crawling stage, second-hand trousers or slacks may be bargains. Equally, children with braces will wear through fabric continuously, and will need a large supply of sturdy trousers. It is no disgrace to be dressed courtesy of the bargain shop, and it may be a very sensible policy indeed if clothes are to be quickly ruined. It is in any event much better to buy old clothes and feel happy for a child to spill paint, play in water, and generally explore in them, than to spend an inordinate amount of money on beautiful clothes, which then have to be guarded (along with their wearer) against any messy experiences.

Underwear

Children suffering from incontinence will need to wear special under-garments (see section on incontinence beginning on page 66). They may prefer to cover these pants with normal cotton or nylon under-pants: This gives added protection and warmth and also helps to avoid the crackling sound which many plastic pants make after a few washes. Underwear generally needs to be warm, and undershirts are easiest to put on if they have wide necks and/or fasten in front. There is a wide range of normal underwear for the under-fives which is perfectly suitable. Older children may like thermal underwear, which is light but exceedingly warm and which has the advantage of not retaining moisture. Easy evaporation of perspiration can be a problem if a child gets very hot propelling a wheelchair or using crutches, and this thermal underwear is particularly suitable for the purpose. In hot weather, pure cotton is preferable to synthetic fabrics.

Adolescent girls have special problems with underwear. Back-fastening brassieres can be difficult to do up, although the sub-sitution of broad elastic so that the garment can be put over the head then pulled into place may help. It is also possible to buy combined bra-slips, which simplify dressing. Although it is possible to buy tights with open inserts, they are not very suitable for many wheel-chair children because of the difficulties in adjustment. Stockings may prove more acceptable, with the old-fashioned garter belt; and socks may be a convenient alternative under long skirts or trousers. Socks and stockings, however, both need to be chosen with some care. If they are made of stretch nylon, they will give a close and attractive fit. But the tops of the socks or stockings may compress the leg and possibly cause circulation or pressure sore problems. If a child has to wear braces, socks are cosmetically attractive. But because they are stretched more than on an average calf, they give a proportionately greater chance of pressure on the leg. In these cases, attractive knitted leg warmers or knee socks may be a practical alternative. It is also possible to buy tubular socks without a fixed heel. These are very easy to adjust.

Indoor Clothes

Most wheelchair children normally find it easier to put on their clothes in two halves, so separates are to be preferred over one-piece clothes. It is also often possible to modify clothes to suit the needs of severe handicaps by adding additional openings: Boys may need zippers or velcro fastenings inside trouser legs (especially if they wear a urine-collection device) or down the back of a coat or in its sleeve; girls may find that elastic waist or wraparound skirts are best. Both sexes may find track suits comfortable; they are stretchable, frequently have inside leg zippers, and are cheerful and light. Care needs to be taken, in the selection of any garments, to ensure that they are comfortable in a wheelchair. A child with scoliosis (curvature of the spine) may find a conventional placement of the waist uncomfortable. A child who has to lean forward to work at a desk or table may have a continuous gap between top and bottom clothes because of the posture he needs to adopt. A tunic top, pinafore dress, or a strip of velcro to hold top and trousers or skirt together, may solve the problem. If a child wears a urine-collection bag, because of the urinary diversion, there may be problems with skirts and trousers that rest on the hip rather than on the waist. If clothes press on a bag, they may kink it or cause leakages. If a girl with a urinary device wears a short dress, it is recommended that a matching cover for the bag may be made so that it bends with the dress.

Outdoor Clothes

Wheelchair children will need more protection than ambulatory children in bad weather. Heavy coats and jackets are restricting in a wheelchair, so a lightweight parka may prove the best choice. Girls often like to wear capes, but care should be taken that the slits are correctly placed for the arms to extend to push the wheels: Slits can be lengthened if necessary. In mild weather, crocheted or knitted ponchos are often enough. But warm gloves and socks are important. It is sensible to tape the former, and either thread them through the jacket sleeves, or provide loops to fasten to the wheelchair or wrist. Pushing wheels is hard on the wrists of clothing, and gauntlet-style gloves or arm-guards are useful (see discussion under Protective Clothing). If a child is going out unaccompanied in a busy street, it may be a good idea to provide a pocket inside one of the outer garments for money and keys, and so forth. Most wheelchair bags hang across the back of the chair, out of the immediate sight of the occupant. In very wet weather, a cycling cape is waterproof and convenient, and can be easily carried in a wheelchair. It is possible to purchase leg muffs which resemble half-size sleeping bags. These zip at the front and offer good protection in very cold weather. Simplantex products produce a wide range of weather wear for wheelchair users. The Wheelymac is an all-in-one waterproof nylon cover with a hood. A wheelchair apron is made of waterproof nylon which covers the user's legs and the wheelchair arms. The "Cosy-Sit" is a quilted foam-lined cover with a woolen lining which zips up, covering the feet and the legs of the user. Comfy Products make the popular "Comfy Cover." This is made of double-thickness silicone-proofed quilted nylon and zips up to waist level like a sleeping bag. Alvema Rehab (Ortho-Kinetics, Inc.) also makes one-piece raincapes for use with their wheelchairs.

Getting Dressed

A wheelchair child with strong arm and trunk control may not have any great difficulty in dressing, provided that suitable clothes are chosen. But a child with poor hand control or balance will need much more skill, and it is useful to ask a physical therapist for suggestions about the easiest method of putting clothes on. Some children will find it easiest to get dressed in bed. Others will prefer to move to their wheelchair. But until a child has mastered dressing skills, it is sensible to provide tough clothes which will withstand pulling and stretching. Stretch fabrics greatly ease manipulation, and velcro fastenings or extra-long zippers will help. Zippers and buttons can be manipulated by tapes or by hooks. Special hooks can be purchased commercially, but are probably best made to suit individual children. Handles can be made out of lengths of broom handle or rubber tubing, and the hook can be made from plastic covered thick wire, or part of a bent coathanger. To avoid difficulties in manipulating buttons, it may be preferable to use elastic-looped buttonholes so that the garment can literally be stretched on and off.

Dressing and undressing is always easier if well-planned. Planning may mean that the parents should sit down and dress *themselves*

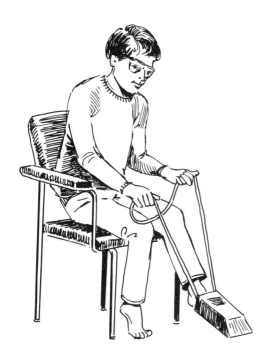

Special aids can be made or purchased to help with dressing. Socks can be pulled on without bending. A stocking "gutter" can be made from a curved piece of plastic or thick cardboard with tapes attached.

in front of a mirror, using clothes of a similar type to those worn by their child. If they observe their own actions, step by step, they will not only be able to break each task down into its separate stages, but to see where particular garments cause problems, and where fastenings might be modified. Children also are often helped by a *large* mirror, so that they can see what they are doing. If two mirrors are positioned so that there is a clear view of the back, it will be much easier to manipulate back fittings with a button hook or similar instrument.

Many garments are difficult to put on simply because they are made of rigid fabric. If a silk or nylon lining is added, or another material substituted, the garment may be much easier to put on or take off. Heavy garments are always difficult to manipulate, because of their weight, but wide sleeves, large armholes, and slippery linings will help. It is therefore important not only to look for clothes which are comfortable and fashionable, but to ensure that they are selected with a view to getting them on. Whenever possible, buttons and other tricky fastenings should be eliminated. Buttons can be left, if ornamental, but the actual means of fastening can be adapted by using elastic on sleeves and velcro on shirt fronts and blouses.

Protective Clothing

Some children with cerebral palsy or a mental handicap dribble a great deal, due to paralysis or malfunctioning of their tongues. Sometimes a speech therapist can counteract this with special exercises to control salivation. If not, some protection will need to be given to clothes. Wool or knitted garments should be avoided because of their tendency to matt and discolor. Their texture will also become harsh unless protected. Bibs can be made of soft toweling or absorbent cotton for young children. But older children will not wish to appear so babyish, and may prefer pinafores, sleeveless overalls, or special bibs made in materials to tone in with their dress or shirt. These false fronts can be made very simply and secured with velcro or tapes. Alternatively, tee shirts or other soft cotton tops or shirts can be worn without special protection and changed frequently. Since drooling or dribbling can produce acute embarrassment, it is worth remembering that darker or bright patterned materials show damp streaks and marks to a lesser degree than plain pale colors.

Children with dribbling problems are also likely to have difficulties in feeding. A wide range of plastic or synthetic painting smocks are available from general stores, and are protective and attractive for meal times. It is obviously preferable to avoid too many changes of clothing during a day, but it is equally wrong for a child to be continually nagged to be careful or, alternatively, to be overassisted in order to avoid mess. Proper protective clothing may in the long run help to prevent overdependency.

Wheelchair girls often like long skirts and dresses. They are warm and cosy and cosmetically attractive if there are lower limb deformities or crutches and braces. It is absolutely essential that these long garments should be made of nonflammable material. Most homes have gas, electric, or open fires. Even if these are protected by fireguards, a child with no sensation in the legs may sit too close or brush against them without noticing the danger. There are a wide range of flame-retardant fabrics on the market. Most garments contain a label indicating the fiber used in manufacture, but older children's garments are less likely to be specifically fire retardant than those manufactured for younger children. If there is any doubt, the buyer in the shop or store should be able to make enquiries from the factory. Attention should also be paid to overgarments, such as ponchos, which may have long fringes hanging over the edge of the wheelchair. These can become caught in the mesh of a fireplace screen or in the spokes of a wheelchair and are a double safety risk.

Children using a self-propelled wheelchair may need special "sleeves" to protect their clothes. A range of painting sleeves are available from toy manufacturers. Alternatively, sleeves can be simply made from an appropriate material. They are simply tubes with elastic ends, which are pulled on and off as necessary. Some children need gloves to protect their hands. Wool or leather gloves may be suitable, but sometimes these are slippery with a poor grip. Gardening gloves, with their cotton backing and soft leather-type palms, are practical and cheap.

If a child has to wear braces or a prosthesis (additional limb), his sensitive skin may need some protection from the appliance. Tubular stockingettes can be purchased and can be cut to size to fit under an appliance. If a child wears an upper limb prosthesis, it may be more comfortable to fit this over a cotton undershirt. Children who use crutches tend to perspire under the arms, because of effort and pressure from the crutches. Their clothes will need reinforcing and changing more frequently if they are to remain fresh. Soft cotton or other absorbent blouses, shirts, or tee shirts are practical. There is a wide range of brightly colored terry cloth tops, intended for beach wear but attractive and practical for younger children. In addition to its absorbency and thickness, terry cloth has the advantage of being normally manufactured in a stretch fabric for younger children's clothes. It will therefore adapt to limb deformities or braces without risk of tearing.

If a child wears braces, there will probably be excessive wear on certain areas of clothing. A way to overcome unnecessary waste is to sew strengthening patches inside the garments. If these are made of a slippery and smooth synthetic material, the edges of the brace will glide over it instead of catching on threads and causing snags and small tears. If stitching patches will spoil the appearance of the garment, there are a number of iron-on patches and tapes which also offer smooth reinforcement. Many iron-on patches, however, tend to become detached at the corners with repeated washings and care should be taken that they do not form rough areas in which the brace will catch. If braces appear to be very rough, or their joints are hard, it is worth asking if they can be covered in soft chamois-type leather. This reduces friction considerably and makes the appliances more comfortable to wear. Whether braces are covered or not, trousers which have to be pulled up over them will wear if the legs are too tightly fitting. Their life will be greatly prolonged either by choosing wider leg fittings (flared legs are particularly convenient) or by the insertion of zippers into the inside lower leg area, as in the conventional track suit. If a child has to wear a hip or waist brace, it may also be necessary to adapt the waist area both by reinforcement with tape or elastic, or by extending the opening area. Skirts will be less likely to be damaged if they are put on over the head and pulled down, rather than lifted up. They are also less likely to be torn if they wrap around and tie, rather than fasten with the conventional button and zipper.

Footwear

Handicapped children need well-fitting footwear as much as their mobile brothers and sisters. Even if a child is confined to a wheelchair, feet can become compressed or distorted by inappropriate shoes. If a child is wearing shoes simply for warmth and appearance rather than practicality, a wide range of comfortable shoes can be purchased in ordinary shops. Children with malformed feet may find open-toed or sling-back sandals, canvas shoes, or baseball shoes comfortable.

Some types of shoes may be difficult for a wheelchair child to put on if he has stiff leg muscles or difficulty in bending. If buckles and laces present problems, they can be replaced with elastic or with elastic laces, so that the shoe is simply slipped on and off. Short sheepskin-lined boots are warm and smart for winter wear, and are easily managed if they have a front zipper. This can be pulled up with a button hook or with a tape. Since in wheelchairs children may tread down the backs of shoes through the positioning of their feet on the chair's footrest, care should be taken that the shoes do not become wrinkled and uncomfortable or actually fall off. If the normal foot position puts undue strain on certain parts of the shoe, the basic shoe shape may be maintained for longer by using shoe trees at night.

When a child is very small, there are a number of soft shoes and boots that are flexible and comfortable and that are available from a range of children's shops. Boots and shoes are easier to manage if they open right to the toe or are elastic. If a child is incontinent and there is frequent staining and soiling of the shoe, cheap canvas shoes can be bought in a wide range of colors. They are easy to keep clean.

LEARNING TO SPEAK

We live in an age dominated by the media—and hence by communication. Language matters and speech delays probably concern parents almost as much as major physical problems. We all know the two- and three-year-old's tantrums for which failure to communicate is largely responsible and that the importance of speech as a key to living cannot be underestimated. Fortunately, perhaps, speech is principally acquired at home. The parent who talks to the child at bath time, plays singing games with him when dressing or feeding, who tells or reads the traditional stories and nursery rhymes, is in fact a teacher. Most children understand a good deal long before they themselves can verbalize that understanding. If they do not understand—because of mental handicap, visual or auditory defects, or lack of stimulation—they will not speak. There are some mentally handicapped children who acquire a "parrot" style speech, memorizing sounds and sentences without any real comprehension of their meaning; but most children will begin by acquiring the sense of a song or sentence before they understand precise meaning. That is to say, the "night-night" or "time for night-night" will signify sleep, the "all fall down" the action of ring-a-rosies. The precision use of words will follow, if the child has an opportunity to hear and repeat a familiar vocabulary. In this context, consistency is important. The child living in an institution who is cared for by a number of care- takers and who has no chance to learn individual word patterns, will be slower to speak than the child who is consistently in the care of one or two grown-ups.

If the child is regularly cared for by people who know and care for him, he will wish to respond to them. His early speech will be sounds rather than words—but his mother will interpret their meaning. If the repetition of a particular sound brings a particular response, it will be repeated and in time polished and amended. But if a child is slow in acquiring understanding, he must be helped.

There is a range of games that encourage the child to recognize and use his knowledge of words. A few small toys in a box or on a tray can be used for "where's the. . .?" If the child recognizes the object, he will be rewarded. Rewards, or reinforcements, need not be candy or even "things." The reward should be praise and delight from the parent.

If speech is difficult for physical or psychological reasons, it is doubly important to show that speaking *means* something. If a mother spends so much time with a handicapped child that she literally anticipates his every need by his facial expression, he will not need to speak. Equally, an overenthusiastic mother may supply such a resounding commentary on the day's activities that she literally leaves no time for the child to get a word in edgewise. Speech is a two-way process, and nursery rhymes, simple games with toys and pictures, and story books are good ways of involving a child's interest. It may be a long time before a child with a severe speech impediment can say "wolf" or "grandma" or indeed comprehend exactly what a wolf is. But he can certainly join in with actions and wolf noises when Red Riding Hood visits the cottage. He can chop with his fingers when the woodcutter comes to the rescue. And he will have learned to follow a sequence of thoughts to a conclusion—which is basically what fiction is all about.

Plainly some parents will be tempted to be overambitious. There are many beautiful—and sophisticated—children's books on the market. But some of these are quite outside the comprehension of a minimal vocabulary. Experiment and try out several books from the local children's library or choose something from the wide range of bright and cheerful paperbacks on the market. If the child has a pet dog or cat, if he likes red balloons or rides in the park, it is not difficult to find subject matter to fit in with his preoccupations. Many children develop obsessions with particular stories; which are read and repeated twenty times and committed to heart before they are cast aside. Repetition ensures that vocabulary is stored and retained in the memory. It is necessary to give the handicapped child an opportunity to hear and inwardly digest what he reads and sees, in the same way as the able-bodied child.

If a child is very slow in learning to talk—or if there appears to be a genuine physical impediment (as in many highly intelligent cerebral palsy children)—the advice of a speech therapist should be sought. Unfortunately, trained speech therapists are in short supply. Although many area health authorities and education authorities employ speech therapists, they are usually overworked and parents may have to help themselves. Although it may be expensive to employ a speech therapist on an individual basis, it is quite possible for a group of parents from a local area to employ a therapist between them.

The success of any speech therapy will, in any event, depend on more than "token" therapy, that is to say, upon one or two half-hour sessions a week. The basic principles will need repeating and reinforcing *every day*. If the parent is to work with her child, it is necessary to be very clear about certain things. First, the child will have to find the experience enjoyable. Second, the parent will have to be determined to find time *regularly* during the day for exercises and practice. Third, that time will have to be when the child is cooperative and other members of the family are not clamoring for attention. Fourth, the precise objects to be achieved should be determined in advance and stuck to. Like playing the piano, speech needs practice and is better learned in short stages. It is much better to concentrate for ten minutes on a particular game or exercise than to spend an interrupted half hour on a variety of activities. Equally it is unrealistic to be overambitious. Success is often gradual and almost imperceptible. Although some children (particularly those whose hearing is discovered to be faulty and is remedied by an appropriate aid) can make miracle breakthroughs, the acquisition of speech is a time-consuming process. For ideas on developing games and activities that encourage speech, *Let Me Speak* and *Let Me Play* (Roy McConkey and Dorothy Jeffree, Souvenir Press, London), cannot be bettered.

Some parents quite innocently *discourage* their children from speaking by anticipating every need and gesture. One of the problems of a wheelchair child's life is the physical curtailment of choice. Because he is restricted and may spend a large amount of time with his parents, they and he can become programmed to one another's needs. It may take time and create frustrating scenes when parents first insist that a small child asks for milk rather than points at the table or says what sweater he wishes to put on in the morning. Plainly children should be neither bullied nor forced, but parents should beware of being too protective. When the child moves outside the home more, he will have to speak—or else run the risk of being treated as the proverbial "cripple." And there are tactful methods of persuasion open to parents who feel their child *could* speak more: They can for instance pretend not to understand, rather than confront the child by refusing to accept gestures, grunts, or nods!

Some children may be helped by exciting toys to trigger off the need to speak. Telephones or intercom systems which can be operated in different rooms, cassette recorders, or even talking dolls may all influence a desire to communicate. Vocabulary can also be helped by "labeling" toys and games. Picture dominoes, lotto, simple picture books, or collections of farmyard animals or small dolls are equally useful. Some children respond to simulated household activities in doll houses or with dolls' tea parties. Very many children provide a running commentary when playing with miniature toys, furniture, cars, and so forth. This "symbolic" play encourages them to act out experiences in their own day-to-day lives and hopefully to comment on them. If a child is sensitive about his poor intonation or lack of vocabulary, he may literally close up when an adult is present and urging him to greater efforts. In this case, the company of other children and a more relaxed play situation may encourage him to relax. Play groups frequently encourage children to speak, when a child has previously appeared frozen in a one-to-one situation with an adult whom he is anxious to please.

There is a wide range of small doll furniture and equipment on the market now, in virtually indestructible plastic. Products by Fisher-Price, Play People, Lego, and so on are all useful for storytelling on themes as far apart as the Wild West or going into hospital. A doll's house can be used to teach concepts such as "up and down" or "in and out." Toys of this kind can also be used as a basis for communication with other children. Many handicapped children, because they are slower to develop clear and useful speech, become accustomed to playing in a solitary dream world. Other children can encourage them to extend their own vocabulary and enjoy a social experience. Therefore toys which encourage planning, thinking, and imaginative use of language are all valuable. Many toys can be borrowed on a trial basis from toy libraries or play schools before purchase to see if they meet special needs.

And sometimes toys that are too complex for a handicapped child to handle, such as electric model railways, are in fact good investments because they attract *other* children. Children swarm like bees around the proverbial honeypot to a home where there is an abundance of good toys, paper, paints, and crayons; and physically immobile children *need* friends who will come to them.

Some children enjoy acting, and finger and hand puppets are fun for imaginative play. Finger puppets can easily be made from felt or scraps of material, with faces drawn with felt-tipped pens. Paper bags (never plastic) or cardboard boxes can be painted, holes cut for eyes and mouth, and used as masks. Older children may enjoy dressing-up games, and a trunk of garage sale clothes and hats may be a powerful incentive to neighborhood children to come in and play.

Older handicapped children may have a quite different speech problem. They are lacking neither in the ability to speak nor in basic vocabulary—but because of their own social inexperience and lack of opportunity, they are bad at spontaneous expression. Since casual conversation is the key to new friendships, and probably will contribute to success in any job placement, these children need every encouragement to speak and to vocalize. Some children will enjoy playing with a cassette recorder—particularly if they can record themselves with friends or other members of the family.

Others need social situations—which the parent may have to contrive. The "does he take sugar in his coffee" syndrome is still sadly widespread—many people feel an instinctive anxiety and embarrassment on meeting a wheelchair person; because they are embarrassed, they are gauche; and because to be gauche is to be socially maladroit and know it, they quickly retreat from the situation. Handicapped children should thus be firmly involved in family social occasions as *children.* They should be encouraged to make friends and (where possible) invite them home and visit them in turn.

Many handicapped children, for instance, never have an opportunity to be with a friend alone: At school or on the school bus, they move as a group; at home, their family is always there. But there are a number of clubs and many local youth group which offer an opportunity to mix freely without Mom or Dad.

If a child is very shy, the onus to make social contacts may initially rest with the parents. Nothing is more painful than to feel a "wallflower." Yet the consequences of being unable to enjoy spontaneous social contact are too dreadful to be ignored, so it is worth putting a great deal of effort into encouraging ease of speech and communication. If a child cannot communicate properly, he will become unhappy and frustrated. He will also probably find it difficult to make decisions.

When speech is difficult to understand because of an impediment, the art of gesture can be developed. Articulation is not the only means of communication, but the value of expression and gesture may not be appreciated if social contact is limited to the family setting where everybody *knows* instinctively what the child wants. It is even easy to become so detached from other people that the need to speak is hardly felt at all; You can often see this in large institutions for the handicapped, where the residents sit around in silent and disinterested detachment because there is no motivation to do anything else. Even if diction is very poor and the child liable to receive apparent rebuffs as a result, he should be encouraged to *want* to speak and to do so as much as possible.

4

Living with a Handicap: Problem Areas

No child is an angel all the time. In fact, the handicapped child who is usually well behaved and quiet, who sits neatly in a corner of the room engaged in nothing in particular, could be said to have much more of a problem than the child who is throwing temper tantrums and demanding his own way. With normal children, parents expect to run the full gamut of human behavior, showing interest, pleasure, approbation, criticism, boredom, and downright irritation and anger in varying degrees. But, because both they and the able-bodied children have mobility, they can sometimes avert a head-on collision by simply changing activities, leaving the room, or being diverted by a noise in the street or a suggestion to play in the garden. Parents and handicapped children are in a very different situation. They may suffer from overexposure to one another: It is very difficult to dash out of the room in a wheelchair. It is also very difficult to be distracted, when so much physical effort and forethought are required for very basic activities. In addition, parents may be on their best behavior with the handicapped child. Their own feelings of guilt, sorrow, and desire to compensate for the disability may all outweigh common sense, so that they conceal annoyance or criticism when the expression of these feelings would clear the air.

George Bernard Shaw said that to punish was to injure. In the sense that punishment is often retribution in anger rather than a just reward for misbehavior, he was probably right. Prevention is preferable to punishment, so it is sensible to look at the "trigger factors" for bad behavior. It is very easy to forget, for instance, that children need attention when they are being *good* as well as when they are being naughty. The toddler throwing his plate on the floor to cause a pleasurable stir while his mother clears it up is not very different from the older child throwing a tantrum at bedtime or when it's time for washing the dishes or helping in the house. If a handicapped child is behaving badly—if he creates a scene in the supermarket, or insists on going to bed so late that he destroys the parents' limited opportunity for privacy, it is sensible to look at the total organization of the day. Reinforcing *good* behavior is much more effective than, through inertia, reinforcing *bad*. A handicapped child is particularly vulnerable with regard to unsociable and unpleasant behavior. First, he will, even more than other children, need to be liked and respected. Second, his more restricted physical environment will make him dependent and perhaps slower to acquire the nuances of desirable behavior through observation and imitation. A common phenomenon is the adult in residential care, who has come to accept service as a duty from society, and whose behavior is so dependent that it remains immature and spoiled. This rather sad phenomenon can be avoided. The wheelchair child will rely on his parents' guidance in establishing appropriate behavior patterns.

Many parents of normal children would like to know the secret of coping with the impossible temper tantrums of a two-year-old. Indeed, all children will and should go through periods of independence and rebellion when they will challenge *all* authority, and little children cannot postpone gratification—they are governed by immediate emotion. As normal maturing proceeds, reason begins to govern emotion. It is this period that especially matters for a handicapped child. Most parents will feel very much at a loss when thinking about disciplining a child in a wheelchair: Punishment seems to add insult to injury. But at the same time, consistent bad behavior creates stress and irritation. No one wins in a war of nerves, and the sensible solution to a behavior problem is to consider carefully what is the "trigger factor."

If Judith repeatedly throws her toys on the floor or tears up and destroys books at an age when she should show more responsibility, or if John persists in resisting bedtime with screaming fits, thumping on the wall, and demands to come downstairs, punishment is unlikely to bring much improvement beyond short-term relief for the parents followed quickly by guilt. Punishment in fact, teaches children what *not* to do, but it does *not* teach them how they *should* behave. Most children will respond very readily to reinforcement (or rewards) for good behavior. These rewards need not be tangible objects like candy or comics: They can be time and attention, joining in a game, reading a bedtime story, or making a painting.

If John is difficult at bedtime, it may be that his physical needs have taken precedence all day, and he *does* need some relaxation and fun before he can sleep. Establishing a play time on a regular basis with stories and games may help. Many of us do not really sit down and talk and play with our children. We think we do—but days are busy and fragmented, and attention divided. If John is not feeling unwell or is afraid of the dark, his family can begin to insist that bedtime is absolute and there will be no further social trips down in front of the television.

It is important to remember, when dealing with any behavior problem, that the problem will probably get temporarily *worse.* John will certainly scream and protest more than ever for a few nights. After all, from his point of view he is suffering deprivation. But when routine is established, he will probably settle down. Ignoring a crying child is always difficult. But living with a handicap is difficult too, and it is essential that parents establish a living pattern that gives them some independence and private time too. Most children are quite capable of recognizing fair play, and provided that they do have their special times and treats, they can accept that other members of the family have rights too.

If Judith throws her toys or food on the floor, or if Susan refuses to get dressed in the morning, the same principles apply. Throwing toys, showing destructive behavior, or playing with food may simply be devices to attract attention. If the parent can show pleasure when a toy is played with constructively, or food eaten, or initiate a more creative activity in place of the game or object which excited destruction, the child may quickly take her cue. It is obviously more difficult to enforce or encourage some forms of behavior in a wheelchair child (like picking up scattered toys or mopping up spilled milk), but a child can be asked to remedy bad behavior in various ways. Milk or food can be cleaned up with a long-handled squeegee mop (if this is regarded as a reward, not a punishment, the child can be encouraged to help more generally with housework); toys can be swept up with a broom or one of the long-handled dustpans and brooms. If parents and children get too upset, the child can be taken out of the room for a short time. But ignoring bad behavior is often the most effective treatment; this can be very difficult in a face-to-face situation.

Some children, of course, have problems of hyperactivity and destructiveness as secondary effects of medication, or because of their brain injury or illness. These conditions will be much harder to treat and live with. But it is important to avoid assuming that they are unavoidable. The hyperactive child may need more occupation and involvement. He may equally be reacting against his parents' rigid insistence on certain behavior patterns to which he is incapable of responding. Children need a framework of rules—they can be flexible, but it is important that a handicapped child also learns that there are obligations within the family circle. Brothers and sisters will be very jealous of special privileges, and the handicapped child's place in the family will not be helped or reinforced by spoiling or what appears to be favoritism.

Brothers and sisters, in fact, may themselves develop behavior problems through having a handicapped brother or sister. These problems will be most likely to arise from the mother's preoccupation with the handicapped child, and from feelings of suppressed jealousy. Older siblings will probably feel very guilty about this jealousy of a disabled child—they may be ashamed that they do not help more, and possibly also feel guilty and resentful about having a handicapped brother at all. Adolescents may be reluctant to bring friends home (especially where the handicap is congenital) and inadvertently add to the mother's work by ceasing to be willing to take the child out in the wheelchair or to babysit. It is alarmingly easy to make the unhandicapped child into a second mother; to request household help which would not be required in an able-bodied household. If the mother is afraid that the handicapped child feels isolated and lonely, she may impress upon brothers and sisters that their duty lies with the family. Children may not be allowed to go and play in the street, where the handicapped child will see them and feel envious. Such behavior is well motivated. But it is disastrous. A handicapped child needs his family's total goodwill, and will need it even more with maturity and the lessening capabilities of his parents. Additionally, brothers and sisters are keys to social life of the neighborhood. They can bring normal children into the house. They can familiarize them with the handicapped child, and this can mean invitations and opportunities which it would be otherwise difficult to contrive. If the brothers and sisters seem to be behaving badly, it may simply be that they recognize an unfair division of resources. However unreasonable a parent may feel this to be, they have their needs and rights. Some families solve the difficulty with timetables allocating each child certain periods of the day or weekend for undivided attention. Most families have favored and unfavored chores. Children can be encouraged to select their own areas of interest, and the reward will be time with their parents.

Parents with a handicapped child may have a desperate longing to have another "normal" baby. This feeling in no way invalidates the love they feel for the handicapped child. But the birth of a baby is an enormous domestic upheaval in any household, and the presence of a wheelchair child will make additional heavy demands on the household. A handicapped child may be more jealous than his age would suggest. A "normal," able-bodied baby will seem to him a replacement, and he will certainly notice the time which the mother now has to devote to the baby. This is a point at which brothers and sisters may draw closer, but it is equally a time when they may feel that this is yet another drain on parental time and love. Every family has to determine its own priorities. With a handicapped child it also needs to take a very balanced view of its strengths and weaknesses in undertaking new ventures.

INCONTINENCE

Like sex and death, incontinence represents one of the social taboos in our society. However, while we have come to terms with sex and (to a lesser extent) with bereavement and death, incontinence is still little discussed and rarely acknowledged. Many wheelchair children are not incontinent. But those who are paraplegics or who suffer from the more severe form of spina bifida are likely to have to grow up with this problem. Precisely because incontinence is rarely acknowledged in the media (or indeed as the frequent cause of the institutionalization of an elderly or disabled person), its significance is rarely appreciated by those who do not experience it. Incontinence usually cannot be "cured." In the disabled, it is due to a malfunctioning of the normal body systems for excreting liquid waste (urine) through the kidneys and bladder, and solid waste (feces) through the bowel. This malfunction may manifest itself in many ways. Some severely handicapped people never have the sensation of desiring to empty bowels or bladder. They lack control of the relevant muscles and they may need help not only to make their disability socially acceptable, but in order to maintain health by a regular pattern of excretion. Their parents (in infancy and early childhood) and they themselves (in later life) will have to assume responsibility for functions which the rest of us rarely consider except when we ourselves temporarily malfunction through nerves or illness. However, it is perhaps salutary to reflect that we are all incontinent at the beginnings of our lives! Many of us will be again at the end, and we need to believe that—even if incontinence cannot be prevented—it can at least be managed in order to enable a child to live a normal social life without undue embarrassment.

Urinary Incontinence

When an able-bodied person needs to empty his bladder, he feels pressure on the urinary tract that encourages him to go to the bathroom. Emptying urine at regular intervals is important to everybody. Urine, which is allowed to collect and distend the bladder, can become stagnant and cause infection. It can also cause back pressure on the kidneys and impede their functioning. Our Victorian forefathers were correct in assuming that several pints of water a day were good for health. Healthy kidneys need fluid literally to flush them out, and more paraplegics will die of kidney infection (caused through bladder problems) than from the direct results of their original injury or disability.

The general aim, in dealing with incontinence, is to try to regularize the passing of urine so that the child can remain dry for reasonable periods of time. This will not, surprisingly enough, be helped by dramatic cutting down on consumption of liquids. Anybody with paralysis *must* ensure that the bladder is fully emptied at least three or four times a day, and the easiest way to ensure this may be to drink a large amount of water. The main drink should be taken first thing in the morning upon wakening, and this can be followed by drinks at regular intervals throughout the day, to serve as "triggers." Although a paraplegic will not experience the normal sensations to warn him that his bladder needs emptying he can usually produce a reflex action to persuade it to empty at will. Physical therapists can usually advise on the most appropriate action. Tapping or kneading the stomach, pressure on the perineum (the skin area just in front of the bowel opening), or tickling and stroking the thighs work in some people. Others may find that the act of drinking produces peristaltic waves (involuntary movements of the intestines), which in turn encourage the bladder to empty. It is important to establish a regular routine, so that retention of urine for limited periods is possible, because paraplegics *must* drink. Five or six pints a day are not excessive, because the risk of infection passing from the bladder to the kidney is very real. Although antibiotics can be used to treat kidney and bladder infections, they are not often wholly successful, and the start of infection may mean a life-long problem, which will be exacerbated in adolescence, and may be critical (in the case of girls) to any future hope of having children. Naturally, handicapped children—like their able-bodied friends—will sometimes wish to make social outings without having to think about the problem of finding an accessible bathroom. In this case liquid consumption can be cut down for two hours beforehand, but it must be made up on the return home.

If the bladder is not emptied regularly, acute urinary retention may result. Sometimes other physical symptoms precede this condition: Headaches, flushing, sweating, or trembling are common. Since the bladder often learns to respond to a regular routine, these symptoms may be due simply to a lapse in the routine and the bladder should be emptied immediately.

Some children will not achieve any degree of control. If the bladder sphincter (that is, the muscles round the mouth of the bladder) is affected, urine may leak and dribble out continuously. It is not possible to retrain this type of bladder, and acceptable methods must be found to control the leakages. Young children will normally wear incontinence pads or diapers with plastic pants. Some pads are basically the same as disposable baby diapers. For slight dribbling, ordinary sanitary pants and pads can sometimes be used (the pads attach to the pants with self-adhesive spots). One special pad resembles these conventional sanitary pads, but contains a substance that "gels" when wet and absorbs three times as much fluid as the conventional pad of similar size. Pads can be worn with "marathon" or other one-way liners. These diaper liners were invented for babies and filter the urine through to the diaper or pad, leaving the skin dry and clean. They are easily sterilized in conventional powder or liquid diaper disinfectants or by boiling, and are invaluable for preventing skin irritations or rashes.

A wide range of plastic pants is also available. Small children will probably be able to wear conventional disposable diaper pants. These are available with snaps or tie fastenings. Older children can wear pull-on pants (unsuitable for very handicapped wearers), or drop-front or flat-opening styles. Kanga pants (which are unsuitable for double incontinence) are made of the same one-way fabric as marathon diaper liners, and filter the urine through to a pad in a plastic pouch *outside* the pants. Although they need changing frequently to ensure that clothing is not soiled and stained, they are very comfortable for sensitive skin. Many all-plastic pants are highly protective, but extremely hot.

Boys have, in general, less of a problem than girls in managing urinary incontinence. There are a number of body-worn appliances designed for boys and men. These should however never be purchased "over the counter," since accurate measurement and fitting are essential. These appliances fit over the penis like a bag; urine passes from the bag to another bag or container, which is strapped to the leg. It is, of course, quite invisible under a trouser leg.

Both boys and girls can wear Foley (in-dwelling) catheters. Catheters are fine small tubes that are fitted directly into the bladder and are held in place there by a small balloon. Urine drains from the bladder down the tube into a plastic bag. Some of the newer catheters have been left in for some weeks, but the majority are removed two or three times a week. This may be done by a nurse or in the hospital as an outpatient, but many parents can manage to change catheters themselves. This method gives more hygienic control, but cleanliness is absolutely crucial to make sure that no infection goes into the bladder. Because paraplegics lack sensation below the waist, it is also possible for a child to lie or slouch in such a way that the catheter causes pressure, or possibly gets kinked and blocked. Parents need to take responsibility to ensure that urine is collecting in the bag and that it is regularly emptied.

The idea of a catheter may seem frightening, but the lack of sensation in most cases removes any discomfort during insertion or removal, and it offers a reliable method of ensuring dryness. If any of us reflect on our own discomfort on sitting in wet clothes for any period of time, it is not difficult to imagine the discomfort which incontinence pads can cause. Additionally, there is less chance of odor with a properly fitted catheter and bag, and women and men find them aesthetically more pleasing for this reason. An important "plus" for children starting school in "normal" primary schools is that a child may quite easily manage to master the knack of emptying or changing a urine bag. On the other hand, very few young children will be able to change and replace incontinence pads reliably, and this task will be complicated by inexperienced helpers and lack of hot water, privacy, and suitable facilities in the school cloakroom. Children of school age may be acutely embarrassed about their incontinence, and the most convenient and private method possible of coping with it should be devised.

A more dramatic alternative to catheters or pads may be an ileal loop. An ileal loop is an artificial diversion of the bladder through an opening in the stomach wall. The opening, called the *stoma*, discharges urine directly into a changeable plastic bag. This is fitted onto the skin with a special adhesive tape and belt. The advantages of an ileal loop lie principally in the promotion of good drainage from the bladder (particularly important if there is associated kidney malfunction), and a convenient and hygienic method of urine collection. However, ileal loops clearly require parents and children who are able to master the system. And the use of a permanent diversion presupposes access to hot water and a degree of privacy for the child. Otherwise constant problems, both of minor infections and of dependency of the child on the parent, can arise.

Plainly the decision is primarily a surgical one and will normally be made on the basis of the child's overall health and prognosis. Long-term advantages will probably include the body image of the adolescent boy or girl—who may see themselves as more sexually and socially attractive with an ileal loop than with incontinence pads and continual problems of dribbling urine. But the judgment will have to be surgical and social on each case's merits.

Bowel Incontinence

Bowel incontinence is usually less of a problem than urinary incontinence, since there is on average usually only one bowel movement a day. However, failure to control bowel movements may produce acute social distress and severely limit social outings.

Fortunately, even the most severely paralyzed can usually achieve a reasonable degree of bowel control through the adoption of a regular routine. Many people will respond to one or two glasses of warm water drunk immediately on waking first thing in the morning. These can sometimes be combined with glycerine suppositories inserted into the anus to stimulate a bowel movement in ten to twenty minutes. It is not a good idea to take daily doses of laxative without a doctor's advice. Large doses can create a permanent state of irritation in the bowel. They may also make it less likely that the bowel will achieve its own rhythm without medication. Since most laxatives are cumulative, commencement in childhood years may necessitate massive doses in later life.

Although it is generally considered that a regular daily bowel action is necessary, individuals vary greatly in what is normal for them. Normality may vary from several times a day to several times a week. But, when incontinence has been present from birth, it is difficult to know what should be the normal pattern for an individual. A bowel movement cannot be passed until the unabsorbed waste products have arrived in the rectum (the end of the large bowel). When the rectum is sufficiently full, it will normally give signals that it requires emptying. Since these signals will not usually be felt by an incontinent person, the rectum may not (without help) discharge its residue. As more debris is passed down the bowel, it accumulates into a large hard mass. Ironically, this extreme form of constipation may create the symptoms of diarrhea (because of the impacted feces, a liquid discharge seeps past), and the real cause of this more troublesome incontinence may not be appreciated. The anxious mother assures her doctor that the child is not constipated; quite the reverse, and the symptoms are treated rather than the cause.

For this reason, it is worthwhile establishing regular bowel movement and adopting a routine which encourages them. Since psychology plays a part, time and comfort (in a warm, well-heated, and private bathroom) should be allowed. It is useful to allow a child five minutes between hasty dressing, breakfast, and the school bus. If early morning is a problem in a family with a number of children to get off to school, an evening routine may be more conveniently adopted. Professional advice should be sought about the best method to achieve a convenient bowel rhythm. It will help if the mother can note whether any foods produce a natural laxative effect. Some children respond to fresh oranges or other fruits, bran products, or coarse rye bread. It is worth experimenting to find a natural stimulant. Initially a doctor may recommend suppositories or even manual removal of the impacted stools. This can be done quite simply with a gloved finger while the child lies on the bed. Great care must be taken to avoid fissures (tiny cracks or tears) in the interior wall of the anus, either through constipation or through manual removal of feces. These can cause infection and the subsequent development of a fistula which may need surgical treatment.

Because it takes time to achieve a working routine, it is important not to alter this, once established. Changes in routine or in diet may change the pattern of bowel movements dramatically, and reversal may be difficult. A particular problem may be stomach upsets caused by unfamiliar food on vacation or when traveling abroad. If major changes of regime are anticipated, it may be wise to obtain suitable medication in advance. Fortunately, the majority of bowel incontinent children have a tendency to constipation, and can stay clean for several days on end without a bowel movement. Provided that their constipation is not cumulative and the cause of ill health, and that they can produce a bowel motion in an acceptable time and place, their incontinence does not cause major inconvenience or restriction in their lives.

Colostomy

Occasionally abnormalities or disease in the bowel necessitate the creation of an artificial diversion through the stomach wall, to enable the bowel's contents to discharge themselves directly into a special plastic bag. As with the ileal loop, this bag is fastened over the *stoma* or opening with a special adhesive. Colostomies can be efficiently managed if suitable appliances are used correctly and if diet is adjusted to give reasonable control. Although many people are horrified at the prospect of a colostomy, the reality is usually less terrifying if carefully managed.

Personal Hygiene

The mother who described the secret of incontinence management as being a good washing machine was speaking with considerable truth. The socially unacceptable side of incontinence lies principally in the unfortunate connotations of smell and damp linen which accompanied incontinence some years ago. The advent of plastic, or special incontinence pads and pants, and of the various urinary devices, have revolutionized the whole problem. However, all bags need emptying and pads changing at very regular intervals. Skin dampened by exposure to urine needs regular washing and powdering. Many parents forget that minor leakages and spillages are almost inevitable, and unfortunately it is equally inevitable that clothes will smell. This smell will be accentuated by a hot classroom atmosphere, and it is essential for the child's self-respect that he or she has a wide range of washable clothes that can be changed every day.

Well-designed clothes (like wraparound skirts with back openings) will reduce the risk of spillages. If clothes are stained, soaking will remove smell and bacteria. However, care should be taken in the choice of colors and dyes, since most disinfecting and deodorizing powders contain an element of bleach. Boiling kills germs but tends to harden plastic and make it uncomfortable and brittle.

In a small house or apartment, odor may be an extra problem—particularly if a colostomy or more complex bowel routine has to be dealt with. A range of special deodorants designed for hospital use are now available on a commercial basis, including liquid and powder disinfectant or neutralizers which can be added to urine or feces left in a commode or bed pan for any length of time. They are generally less powerfully scented and longer lasting than their commercial equivalents for normal household living. Since any scented product is liable to become associated with what it is meant to conceal, and thus become unpleasant in turn, an alternative may be a small fan in either bedroom or bathroom. These small fans are relatively cheap and can be simply installed by a local electrical business. They can (particularly in winter) be a pleasanter solution than open windows or lavish use of aerosol sprays.

MENSTRUATION

Physically handicapped girls have an additional problem in personal hygiene—the management of menstruation. In certain conditions (particularly spina bifida), the onset of puberty may be advanced by some years into primary school age. Although such cases are rare, the chance of an abnormal pattern should be noted and the child properly prepared. Many parents are reluctant to raise the question of puberty (and its connotations of sex and procreation) with a physically handicapped girl, because they feel it is unkind to emphasize her own difference from her able-bodied peers. However, precisely because a handicapped girl will have less casual access to journals, shops, and a wide range of girls of similar ages, she may have no idea of what is happening to her and be terrified and embarrassed by a normal physical process.

Many adolescent girls experience problems in the early years of menstruation, and very heavy periods may be particularly disastrous for a wheelchair girl, so if there is a real problem, the doctor may be able to prescribe hormone treatment which will regulate the condition. This will normally be provided after referral to a gynecologist.

There is a wide range of pads and pants on the market, and it will probably be necessary to experiment. Many girls will find it difficult to manipulate the conventional belt and pad, and may prefer the more recent developments of pants and pads with self-adhesive patches. These are not suitable for incontinent girls who have not had the ileal loop division, and in the case of incontinence it may be preferable to use internal tampons provided that there is sufficient finger control to manipulate them.

Every effort should be made to emphasize the normality of menstruation. Many able-bodied girls show reluctance to undertake physical activities during menses and feel generally unwell and depressed simply because it is part of the cultural pattern of their families. But care can be taken to avoid the impression that one is bound to feel abnormal or incapacitated at these times. Wheelchair living is sufficiently complex without added fears and stresses.

Since wheelchair girls represent a cross section of the population as a whole, some will of course suffer from premenstrual tension and possibly fluid retention. A few will suffer from physical discomfort, low back aches, or stomach aches. If there appears to be a marked pattern of physical symptoms during the monthly cycle, it is worth consulting the family doctor. Although premenstrual tension is probably less common in its acute form than old wives tales would indicate, there is medical evidence that some women are more accident prone and generally function at a lower level during these few days. If a girl has severe physical discomfort, cramps, or pain, and is already receiving medication, it may be prudent to ask the doctor to recommend a suitable pain killer. But the overall emphasis should be, wherever possible, on normality and acceptance, backed up by full explanation of the developments to be expected.

GOING INTO THE HOSPITAL

Hospitalization is a traumatic experience for all children. For handicapped children, it can be a double disaster. First, a child with a physical handicap is far more likely than others to have *long* periods of hospitalization in early childhood, whether for corrective orthopedic surgery, treatment of Stills disease or hemophilia, or surgical creation of urinary diversion. These periods of special surgery may also mean (as in the case of a child with paraplegia) long-term admission to an adult ward, which may be far from ideal for the emotional needs of the child.

Second, physically handicapped children are more likely to be admitted to special hospitals which are some distance from their parents and friends. This means that visiting may be sporadic and expensive, and parents will be less likely to be able to "room in" with their child or to be relaxed and optimistic when they are visiting.

Third, a handicapped child may have special problems of dependency on his parents. Precisely because his environment has been restricted, he will be accustomed to a limited family circle and routine. The transition to the kind but dispassionate hospital ward may be very frightening, and the resulting emotional problems considerable.

Illness of some kind is a universal stress in childhood, and the "normal" child too is likely to have accidents or illnesses which necessitate brief hospitalization. But whereas the pattern of acute hospital admissions is changing, with early release in the post-operative period and home nursing support becoming more common, children with handicaps face a reversal in the general situation. They are the ones who are most likely to have long stays in the hospital. Yet they are also the ones particularly vulnerable to the emotional problems of separation from their families and from possible painful, certainly uncomfortable, ward procedures. In addition, their adjustment to the new world on the ward will be considerably inhibited by the physical restraint imposed by any orthopedic surgery. Immobile in plaster, on traction, resting in the convalescent period of hemophilia or Stills disease, these children cannot explore and investigate their world. They can only play with the limited toys to which they have access in bed. If the ward is short-staffed, the work of caring for severely disabled children will probably take precedence over play, stories, and personal relationships that are vital to confidence and happiness in the young child.

In a majority of hospitals, mothers can stay with their young children at least through the day, possibly by night as well. This shared care ensures that the child's home routine is not entirely shattered by the hospital, and that the mother does not feel excluded from treatment. But hospitalization for some weeks is a different matter, and many mothers will be visiting infrequently.

But if it is really impossible to visit frequently, there are ways of keeping in touch. Children can enjoy family photographs—these can be renewed from time to time with snapshots of the family dog or guinea pig, the child's room, and so forth. Some children express great anxiety that their room will not be waiting for them when they come home. Needless to say, their belongings and room should remain sacrosanct. Many adults feel unwanted and rejected when they are ill and in the hospital—the child is acutely conscious of his temporary exclusion from home and family and needs a reassuring knowledge of his "other" world.

If a child cannot get to the telephone, he may be able to use cassettes for a two-way conversation. Some hospitals do not like radios or tape recorders, but may compromise if an ear plug is used. The cassette has the advantage of offering the fabric of family life, the dog's bark, the children's voices, maybe Granny sending her love. If a pay phone is available (most likely for a child on an adult ward), a good supply of coins should be left. Few children can manage reverse charges. Letters and post-cards should be sent frequently. If a parent suspects that nobody on a busy ward has much time for reading correspondence to a child who cannot read himself, the letters can be visual. Cut-out pictures, drawings, and pressed flowers can be put on to prepunched paper, which can then be stored in a clip file. Drawings to color in or puzzles can be sent in the same way. Children need to be kept in touch with their home, and lots of letters, pictures, and cards will help when visiting is difficult.

If there is no recreation director on the ward, most children will welcome a good supply of crayons, pencils, paper, clay, weaving, or simple modeling kits suitable for use in bed. Little figures like the play people mentioned in Chapter 11 are suitable for use on a hospital table, and magnetic board games may amuse some children. Fuzzy felt pictures can be bought cheaply and, with gummed paper shapes and jigsaws, offer opportunities for design making and story telling. However, anything with a large number of pieces is liable to get lost, so a suitable storage bag (like a bicycle bag) may be a good idea. Equally, in a ward with a major emphasis on cleanliness and order, messy occupations like modeling clay and cutting out may not be encouraged. A little market research is useful in advance to make sure that gifts are not just tidied away. If the child is old enough to attend school, the hospital teacher can often give practical advice on toys and leisure activities, as well as provide educational instruction. Once a child is allowed out of bed, he will usually have a choice of recreational activities.

If he is bed-bound for a long period of time after surgery, real imagination may be needed to find an occupation. Some children enjoy learning to knit or crochet—sewing is rarely popular with the nursing staff because of the lost needle in bed. Stamp albums and other small items interest some children—and it is worth encouraging these portable occupations if it is likely that there wll be repeated hospital admissions. One grandmother provided a miniature. Japanese garden, with tiny plants, a little lake made from a looking glass, and a tiny path made from gravel. Her grandchild looked after the garden with a doll's watering can and fork. A variety of small ferns and plants can be grown in shallow plastic or china bowls or troughs, including mustard and lettuce, one or two pea plants; acorns, apple seeds, and peach pits can be experimented with. The important thing is to find something of lasting interest.

Particularly if a child is in a distant hospital, where parents cannot visit very frequently, there may be communication difficulties between the parents and staff. Most people are basically frightened and insecure when confronted with the hospital hierarchy. Most of us were nervous around doctors and hospitals when we were young, and we may also have secret fears that any criticism or questioning may affect the treatment of our child. But it is important to establish good lines of communication as early as possible, and most hospital workers will welcome a friendly relationship with parents of children in their care. The head nurse on a ward is of course the logical person to discuss any problems with, but nursing staff operate on shifts and they also come and go. Trainee nursing staff, in particular, change frequently, and parents may not see the same nurse twice if they visit infrequently. So an important person can be the recreation director. On questions about the child's treatment, the recreation director will need to advise parents to talk to the doctors or nurses and for other problems the social worker may need to be brought in. But the recreation director is often well placed to discuss with parents their anxieties about leaving a young child in the hospital for the first time. He or she can encourage parents to help sustain the child's bond with them by providing him or her with information about their home life, and by leaving behind with the child physical reminders such as a familiar possession. It may sometimes be necessary for the director to encourage the parents to visit more frequently if possible and to explain why their child is uninterested or cries and is upset when they see him and why, nevertheless, he needs to see them if he is not to feel abandoned.

Clinging and difficult behavior are particularly distressing to families when a child is in the hospital. Some parents are reluctant to visit because of the storms of tears, rudeness, or lack of interest that confronts them. Older children may be very anxious about other children they see. Maybe a child has died or is so grossly handicapped that it appears nothing can be done for him. The handicapped child may look at himself and for the first time think "Who will look after me when Mommy and Daddy die? Will I live in hospital? Will I get worse like him?" A sensitive child may feel very worried about other children who are not visited, but at the same time resentful of the unvisited child who tries to share *his* visitors and treats. He may also worry about the home and family forgetting him, about his treatment and drugs, and about the surgery itself. Many children are frightened of anesthesia; it symbolizes "going away" as completely as death, and they are worried that they will not wake up again. Many physically handicapped children are hospitalized for orthopedic treatment, and will wake up to a heavily bandaged or plastered limb, so that the improvement—or otherwise—will not be seen for some weeks to come. One small boy was terrified by the janitor's perfectly innocent joke that "he didn't have a real leg in there; they had taken it away in the night." Fortunately the nurse and the hospital recreation director recognized his distress and were able to reassure him. But some children will never admit such fears and continue in extreme anxiety. Many of these problems will be exacerbated by the fact that the child is literally caged in his cot or bed, perhaps in traction or in plaster, and so severely restricted in movement or activity. Some children in this situation become champion throwers or hitters, tossing fruit bowls, toys, or glasses at staff or visitors, or hitting and pushing. Such behavior is not "naughty" in the sense that the child can help it, and is a desperate cry for help. Bad behavior is often intensified when the child first returns home and remembers all that he has experienced—and all that he has lost. This bad behavior is a perfectly natural reaction to a child's hospital experience and is indeed better than total withdrawal and apathy. However, it is difficult to live with, particularly since a wheelchair child is very likely to return from a period in an orthopedic hospital with a leg in plaster or with other physical constraints still operating.

Since his discharge may put additional burdens on the mother—who suddenly has to cope with an immobile, clinging, and naughty child—it is absolutely essential to get as much help as possible. If the recreation director in the hospital has developed interests and skills in the handicapped child during his stay, it is worth noting what activities were enjoyed and reintroducing them at home.

Parents may think they cannot win in the hospital situation: Their child needs specialized treatment, they cannot live in the hospital, and they have all the additional anxieties and stresses to cope with. The important thing is to ensure that the child is frequently visited, that he does have adequate toys and reading and writing material, and that the parents and staff can have a frank and supportive relationship. It is easy to leave comments until they become major complaints, which leave the staff and the parents in permanent confrontation.

SPECIAL MEDICAL PROBLEMS ARISING FROM HANDICAP

Pressure Sores

Handicapped children get ill and have accidents like all children in our society. But they also have some special problems if they are wheelchair bound. Perhaps the biggest problem for the child with paraplegia or severe immobility is the pressure sore. If a child sits in one position all day, because he is paralyzed and cannot move, he is putting excessive pressure on one part of his body. If he has no sensation in the lower part of his body, he may not notice that his leg is pressing hard against the seat of his wheelchair, or that the rug or cushion is creased and the crease is pressing into his thigh. A non-paralyzed person moves continually—small movements which for the most part are carried out quite unconsciously. We are probably only aware of these movements when we "fidget" or have an uncomfortable seat. But these movements continuously redistribute our body weights and ensure that we are comfortable. Without the incentive or ability to redistribute weight, it is easy to compress an area of skin. Compression prevents the circulation of oxygen, and the skin tissue then dies. Dead tissue harbors infection and the end product can be an unpleasant ulcer which may take weeks or even months to cure.

The first sign of a pressure sore is a reddening of the skin. All paraplegics should examine their bodies at least once a day for signs of pressure sores. This is probably easiest done in the bath or shower—a large mirror or a wall of mirror tiles will ensure overall visibility. Special hand mirrors on a flexible handle can also be purchased for use in bed. If a red area is spotted, all pressure must be avoided until the color is normal. Bluish-black marks show the second stage of a pressure sore and need *immediate* medical attention and advice.

Pressure sores are most likely to develop on areas like the ankle or thigh, where the bones are very near the surface of the flesh. It is sensible, therefore, to observe carefully how a child sits or lies. Because prevention is always much better than cure, special cushions can be very practical. These distribute pressure from sitting or lying over the maximum possible area, so that blood flow to the tissues is not restricted in any way. Cushions are not a complete answer, and children must be taught consciously to move their positions whenever possible by push-ups with their hands, movements of their back, or any means which redistributes their weight regularly. Parents will have to perform these movements passively if the child is too handicapped or too young to carry them out actively.

Foam cushions are the most popular (and cheapest) and are simply slices of polyester foam suitably shaped and covered. If foam is unsuitable, cushions filled with polystyrene beads (like the bean bag chairs available on the market) may be comfortable. Air cushions are comfortable for some children, particularly if the degree of inflation is controlled by a valve. Their disadvantage is that they can be hot to sit on (being rubber or plastic), and pressure can sometimes be difficult to regulate if the covering is thick. Water cushions are very similar, except that they are of course sealed rather than adjustable. They can be cold to sit on, the converse of the air cushion, because water absorbs heat. This may be an advantage for some users (perspiration can be a problem for wheelchair users), but may give other children cold bottoms. Gel cushions perform the same function and are equally comfortable, but are heavy. Both gel and water cushions must be treated with respect, as accidental pricks or punctures will end the life of the cushion and be exceedingly uncomfortable for the wheelchair user concerned. Air cushions are cheapest to replace, if damage or punctures are a problem. The more a cushion is handled (and the more journeys it makes in car trunks and so forth), the mor it is likely to be dropped or damaged, unless all users are conscious of the need to take care.

The most sophisticated cushion is the electric ripple cushion. Ripple cushions are air cushions with a difference, since a battery-powered pump and valve system rhythmically inflate and deflate a series of interlinked inflatable tubes, so that the cushion is constantly "rippling" and avoiding any pressure on a particular part of the body. The ripple cushion is not suitable for every child, and medical advice should be sought about its use. However, as with many aids, trial and error is usually the best method of selection. It is often possible to borrow cushions on a trial basis to assess their suitability. The best protection (since no cushion will protect a thigh against a pen dropped down the side of a wheelchair or a knee pressed against a table leg) is constant vigilance. If a child needs lifting and moving at night, it may be possible to extend the principle of the ripple cushion and obtain a ripple mattress, which will ensure that there is gentle and continuous movement. Getting up several times in the night is hard work for tired parents, and children cannot be allowed to turn or exercise their own muscles without supervision. A special bed can help solve this problem for some families.

Because a particular problem with children is often their understandable desire to carry an accumulation of toys tucked into their wheelchair, an answer to hoarding may be a bag slung over the back of the wheelchair or alternatively a stroller-type bag clipped or buckled onto the side arm. Small children often find it difficult to turn round and lift a bag onto their knees, so a side bag or basket has an advantage. Bicycle shops have a wide range of bags and baskets that can be adapted; tricycle bags and baskets are small enough for junior-sized wheelchairs and little toys. Nobody who has accidentally sat on a model car will doubt their power to injure even the ablebodied, and it may be useful for the child to establish a regular routine of checking the sides of his chair and cushions for small toys. If a child who is liable to get pressure sores also wears a safety harness or carries crutches in his wheelchair, care should be taken that they do not press on or contract his limbs.

Some parents are convinced that they will harden their child's skin if they give regular alcohol rubs or massage it liberally with cream or talcum powder. In fact, massage does not help blood to circulate to the skin and actually encourages sores to form. Cleanliness from daily baths, showers, or wash-ups, with conscientious drying before the application of talcum powder is quite sufficient.

If pressure sores happen—despite precautions—it is sensible to get medical advice immediately. The main treatment will be time and avoiding pressure on the area. This may be difficult with a young child, who is reluctant to sleep on his left rather than his right side in bed, or who may not remember the need to keep his feet in a certain position. His parents may have a major supervisory job, and if this is too difficult, hospitalization may be necessary. Usually, however, treatment can be carried out at home.

Because treatment of pressure sores is such a protracted procedure, parents should not trust their children to carry out their own checks. Invasion of privacy is never welcome, but inspection should be insisted upon until the child is clearly competent and able to look after himself. If he is at a special school, self-care will play an important part in his day, and there will be a double check.

Burns and Scalds

All children in wheelchairs are particularly vulnerable to burns and scalds. First, they are, of course, less mobile than normal children, and more liable to catch accidentally against lamps, brush against fires, or manipulate saucepans clumsily in the kitchen. Second, many wheelchair children lack sensation in some of their limbs, and may be quite unaware that they are sitting too near a fire or against a radiator, or that their hand is resting against a hot coffee pot on the table. Thus great care should be taken to see that a child understands the need to be careful. Additionally, sunburn is a very real risk, since skin may be more susceptible over the paralyzed areas, and it is very easy to overdo exposure.

The wheelchair itself is a clumsy object, and the presence of a young child in a wheelchair in the average small suburban apartment or house may be a considerable safety hazard for other children as well as its occupant. If the wheelchair occupies most of the floor width in a narrow kitchen, for instance, other children may be brushed against saucepan handles on the stove or trip and drop a kettle of hot water. Trailing electric cords are a major safety hazard, since they can easily twist around a wheelchair's wheels and pull lamps, toasters, or other equipment to the floor. Since most wheelchairs are lower than work surfaces in an ablebodied kitchen, there is the added risk of the wheelchair child reaching up and knocking equipment over.

Prevention is always better than cure. Fire screens hooked to the walls over any kind of open fire and saucepan guards on the stove to prevent pans accidentally being pulled over are sensible precautions. Additional safety precautions include never allowing the child to get into a bed with the electric blanket on if he is incontinent or has a hot water bottle. It is also very dangerous to carry hot dishes or drinks in a wheelchair—if they must be carried, they should be carried with one hand over the side of the chair in a suitable basket or container. Hot things should never be held over the knees or legs. If small children can crawl or roll around the floor—perhaps on a wheeled crawler—great care should be taken to see that any hot pipes are covered or boxed in, and that they cannot slip against hot radiators. Some oven doors get uncomfortably hot and, although quite safe inasmuch as a child cannot easily open them, are dangerously hot for a paralyzed limb to rest against. Children, of course, have to acquire their own survival code. But they will need watching initially to avoid unnecessary accidents. Burns and scalds, even minor, should always be taken seriously, and receive proper medical attention.

Respiratory Tract Infections

Although—and partly because—propelling a wheelchair is hard work, and the chair's occupant often feels very warm, many wheelchair users are considerably more exposed to extremes of temperature than their able-bodied counterparts. A wheelchair user is unlikely to make the constant involuntary movements necessary to maintain circulation, and may (without realizing it) get very cold. This is particularly true outdoors when watching a game or window shopping. Unfortunately, very heavy clothing does not go easily with the self-propulsion of a wheelchair, but care should be taken to protect paralyzed limbs with rugs or additional warm socks and fur-lined boots in cold weather. It is not uncommon for paraplegics or spina bifida children literally to get frost bite!

Coughs and colds are common hazards of childhood, but again, physically handicapped children can be particularly at risk from chest infections. Their limited physical activity may make it difficult for them to clear their bronchial tubes of any mucus. If the mucus blocks and irritates the linings of the bronchial tubes, infection can result. Cough medicines may offer temporary relief, but do not solve the problem because they merely offer short-term relief from the irritation. If a sedative cough mixture is used, it may even aggravate the infection, because the urge to cough is diminished and the mucus is therefore allowed to accumulate. Because some handicapped children appear to have a predisposition to more respiratory tract infections than their able-bodied brothers and sisters, it is necessary to devise methods of clearing the lungs. Some children need postural drainage. Postural drainage can be simply demonstrated by a physical therapist and is a way of tipping the child and percussing (tapping) his back or chest in order to drain the chest cavity. If this is done regularly, there is little risk of major blockages and infection. The latter is particularly worrying if the child is tetraplegic or severely affected by spina bifida so that his muscular control of the trunk of the body is poor. Many paraplegics are more prone to pneumonia, and special care is needed. Antibiotics may be used with caution in many cases.

Epilepsy

Epilepsy can be described as recurrent seizures or lapses of consciousness produced by a sudden discharge of electrical activity in the nerve cells of the brain. Estimates of the incidence of epilepsy vary from eight to twenty cases per thousand population. The more dramatic *grand mal* seizures are instantly recognizable, but *petit mal* epilepsy may be mistaken for daydreaming or inattention. A diagnosis may be made only after an electroencephalogram reveals the lesion which is the cause of the problem. The electroencephalogram is obtained by placing small plates (electrodes) over the scalp. These electrodes are wired to a machine which records the electric activity in the brain and reveals any abnormalities. The location of the lesion (scar) in the brain which is the focus for the abnormal electrical activity will determine the degree of severity of the epilepsy.

Despite the stigma which is still attached to it, epilepsy is usually completely controllable by anticonvulsants. However, the side effects of the drugs can in themselves cause problems. Some children become sleepy and slow, and their performance at school suffers. The prescription of the correct medication and decision on appropriate dosages should be made by a pediatrician or neurologist and be constantly reviewed. If a child appears to be oversedated or underachieving, further investigation should be considered.

Epilepsy in physically handicapped children is usually a side effect of their handicap—treatment can be more complex in, for example, hydrocephalus where there may be intermittent high pressure in the head through temporary malfunctioning of the drainage valve or through other abnormalities. But most epileptic seizures are of short duration and are due to failure to take the regular medication, high temperature in sudden illness, or the temporary "trigger factor" of a flickering television screen (for those who are photosensitive to flickering lights) or occasionally through emotional problems or early menstruation in young adolescent girls. If a child has a *grand mal* seizure, his condition may appear very frightening. He may bite his lips so that they bleed, froth at the mouth, and twitch. If he is standing up, he will fall down and possibly bang his head or hands in falling. On recovery he may vomit or wet himself. However, the physical symptoms are usually more frightening than the reality. The best treatment is to turn the child onto his side (or turn his head to the side and down if he is in a wheelchair), loosen tight clothes, and wait. The old belief that a ruler or stick should be thrust between the teeth is wrong. Bitten tongues will heal—broken teeth will not!

Normally a child will come out of a seizure in between five and ten minutes. He may be dazed and confused for rather longer and should certainly not be allowed out on his own until he is completely recovered. Some children respond to a glucose drink, others to a short bed rest.

If a child does not recover from a *grand mal* seizure, but goes from one seizure to another without regaining consciousness, it should be regarded as an emergency. The best treatment is immediate transfer to a hospital emergency room, where there will be a range of remedies available. If a private car is available, and it is possible to take the child safely, it should be used in preference to an ambulance to save time. If a child enters into "status epilepticus" (that is to say, into a period of prolonged convulsions), there is a very real risk that he may suffer permanent brain damage. Immediate treatment is almost always effective.

A child's social life may be seriously affected by epilepsy, not because he is necessarily particularly at risk or handicapped by it, but because friends, schoolmates, and relatives are frightened. A child with epilepsy should *always* carry a medic-alert bracelet. This will ensure that if he should have a serious seizure and be admitted to the hospital, there will be no delay in determining the treatment he has been undergoing. If a child is very liable to seizures, he may need to wear a protective helmet. A young child with periodic seizures may need a harness in his wheelchair to make sure that he does not fall forward and hurt himself.

In adolescence, epilepsy very occasionally appears to get worse because the child—through emotional difficulties—is not taking his medication and is actually inducing the seizures. Although this is very unusual, it should be considered if previously well controlled epilepsy reappears. Sometimes children are reluctant to take medication in front of teachers and fellow pupils, and tactful enquiries should be made at school.

Kidney and Bladder Infections

Any child with a spinal cord lesion (as in paraplegia and spina bifida) is likely to have problems with urine incontinence. The bladder can be damaged in two ways. It can lack the muscular tone to empty itself of urine completely, which means that dribbling of urine and infection can occur; or if the *sphincter* muscle at the exit point of the bladder is too tight, it may also prevent the urine flowing easily out into a tube, the *urethra*, which guides urine out of the body. If this is the case, the bladder and *ureters* (the two elastic tubes that lead from the kidneys to the bladder) will fill up and be distended with urine. The enlargement of the ureters can compress the kidneys and damage their filtering mechanisms. If the kidneys fail to operate properly, waste products are not filtered out of the blood but circulate through the body. It has been estimated that the rate of urinary infection in spina bifida children is as high as 90 pecent by eight years old, so it is obviously important to make sure that any infection is treated *immediately* before it affects the kidneys. Some hospitals carry out routine urine tests and special kits are available for home testing. Pus and organisms will be visible under a microscope long before the physical feelings of fever or pain are felt by the child. Treatment is usually by antibiotics and sometimes by antiseptic washouts of the bladder. But unfortunately many children quickly become resistant to the range of suitable antibiotics. Prevention is therefore much better than an uncertain cure.

Prevention can be achieved, first, by ensuring that the child has plenty to drink. In hot weather, the daily consumption of fluid should be increased to allow for perspiration. The paraplegic will not experience warning signals and may neglect to stimulate the reflex action for the bladder to empty itself (see page 68). If a child is incontinent, it may also not be noticed that the bladder is actually storing the bulk of the urine and expelling only the overflow, so it is very important for parents to *check* that their child *does* attend to his bladder at two or three hourly intervals—however engrossing the play activity.

If a child gets a urine or kidney infection, the first symptoms may resemble those of a cold. He may look feverish and irritable. His nose may feel blocked, he may perspire and even vomit, and medical attention is necessary. Sometimes these symptoms, however, are not due directly to infection but to acute urinary retention: The bladder has not been emptied regularly and has become distended, so the immediate treatment is to ensure that the bladder is emptied. If this is not possible, a doctor must be called to empty the bladder through a catheter (a thin tube). If there are obvious symptoms of kidney or urinary infection, he may insert a tube called a Foley catheter. This fine tube has an inflatable balloon at the bladder end, which is inflated in the bladder.

Kidney and bladder infections are rarely entirely preventable— but every effort should be made to ensure that they are avoided as much as possible. If they prove particularly persistent, the hospital consultant may recommend the creation of an *ileal loop* diversion.

Fractures

Children with paraplegia or spina bifida run a greatly increased risk of breaking bones, compared with their mobile brothers and sisters. Due to paralysis, circulation in their legs is sluggish and the bones do not receive the necessary nourishment they need. Because they are thin and brittle, they can be snapped easily, particularly if the child has spent a protracted and inactive postoperative period in plaster. Although many parents feel convinced that their child is *more* likely to have an accident if he tries to walk with braces and parallel bars, the converse is true. Once the circulation is improved by regular exercise, the bones will become stronger and fractures less likely.

If a spina bifida or paraplegic child fractures a bone, he may not realize that anything has happened. A normal child will feel extreme pain and swelling. His strong muscles may pull the two parts of the bone out of position and the break will therefore have to be immobilized in plaster to ensure a good join. The paraplegic cannot feel the painful sensation of the fracture, and the first symptom may be a firm hard swelling on the leg. Because the muscles are not strong, there is little pull on the fractured bone, and it will not suffer much displacement, so there will not usually be any need to set the bone with plaster of Paris splints. Since the skin on paralyzed legs is very sensitive to pressure and to sores (and plaster of Paris is, in any event, difficult to use), treatment will usually be limited to rest and the avoidance of crutches or braces until the fracture has healed. The best prevention is exercise—if walking in braces is impossible, the child's limbs should be gently exercised either by the parents or by the child itself to ensure that the muscles are kept in good order and that circulation is adequate.

Contractures and Spasms

Many people have the inaccurate belief that lying still and "resting" is a proper activity for a handicapped child. While handicapped children, like everybody else, will need to rest when tired and to immobilize limbs which have been hurt in an accident, it is most important that they do not simply lie around unnecessarily. Joints need to be moved through their full range of movement every day. Normally a physical therapist will demonstrate how to do this— since hard pulling and tugging are not useful or comfortable. But if joints are not moved (even if they have no spontaneous movement in them), they run the risk of fixed deformities which will increase with time. The reason for these deformities is that when some of the muscles which move a joint become paralyzed, the joint itself becomes very stiff and "locked" because of its lack of movement. If this stiffness is not dealt with, contractures result. These are literally shortenings of the muscles, and the joint will get increasingly stiff. Eventually it may be impossible to move it at all.

Children can be encouraged to take active exercise (where there is sufficient muscle power to move the limb on its own) or passive exercise (when the paralyzed muscle is manually moved). A wheelchair child may be able to exercise his own legs with his hands. Unless there are medical reasons for not doing so, he should also be able to keep his spine flexible by bending and stretching. This is often done without any special exercise, because the child is playing, picking things off low shelves, or simply manipulating his clothes in dressing. If, despite exercise, a contracture is severe and the tissues around a joint become deformed, it may be necessary to take further action to prevent the joint becoming severely incapacitated. If there is no feeling in the joint (as in the case of paraplegia), great care must be taken not to cause pressure sores or to damage the skin. Strapping or splints are often recommended. The latter can be made of a variety of materials, including leather, fiber glass, and polythene, and are usually fastened with velcro or similar simple fastenings. Care should be taken to use them according to instructions and to make sure that skin care is adequately supervised. Skin damage can result from a few moments' negligence—and ulcers or sores can take months of inactivity to heal. If a child has a fixed deformity (probably through a congenital disability), the physical therapist may teach the parents how to manipulate the deformity to correct it by gradually stretching the tight structures. This manipulation may have to be followed by strapping. Because strapping inevitably involves a tight application of bandages with the corresponding risk of damage, great care should be taken to follow instructions and inspect the skin areas daily.

If deformities result and cannot be resolved through physical therapy, orthopedic surgery may be necessary. Orthopedic surgery is, naturally, a specialist affair and restorative surgery for spin bifida children in particular has developed considerably in the last few years. In some cases straightening of a joint may actually enable the child to achieve limited walking skills. Postoperative care is important, and physical therapists normally advise on exercises and treatment.

Problems with Hearing and Sight

Unfortunately very few children have only one handicap. Serious handicapping conditions like spina bifida or cerebral palsy are usually accompanied by secondary or more minor handicaps. These secondary handicaps particularly cover defects in hearing and sight, which if untreated may make a child appear far more severely handicapped than he really is. Most hospitals now routinely check sight and hearing of any handicapped child, and the majority of child welfare centers also routinely check for defects in all babies. Unfortunately, it is very easy to miss minor deficiencies in hearing and seeing in young children, and parents should ensure that they do no pass over any hearing or sight loss because they feel the child is "just a bit slow."

The majority of children with hearing problems are not totally deaf, so response to your slamming a door or saying "boo" is not an indication of a level of effective hearing. Children may respond to some sounds because of "visual" cues such as seeing their mother's mouth move; or they may very often hear only high or low frequencies. This means that they get a very distorted picture of the sound of words, and their speech and spelling will be severely affected. Even babies can wear hearing aids, and it is important that children should start as early as possible. Usually hearing aids will only be issued after detailed assessment by an audiologist, a specialist in hearing, who tests the child's hearing with special instruments to indicate which tones are picked up and which are missed.

Needless to say, a hearing aid once prescribed should be regularly worn. Deaf children can become very disturbed if there is no adequate means of communication with the outside world, and any hearing problem can be a major cause of apparent educational retardation if it prevents communication. If a child can hear certain tones, but not others, he may give the impression of hearing adequately but will in fact be missing much of what is said. Many handicapped children have high-pitch or tone deafness only, because the cochlea (the spiral of the inner ear) which controls high tones is the most easily damaged. This means that vowels may be heard accurately but not consonants. If diagnosed in time, selective frequency hearing aids can be obtained or (in some cases) the child can learn to lip read to augment his basic hearing, or even learn signing.

Visual handicaps are often no different from those experienced by able-bodied children. However, crossed eyes or other visual deficiencies need to be corrected as quickly as possible. A handicapped child sitting in a wheelchair will not easily be able to get up

89

close to the interesting objects in his environment, nor will he necessarily be able to get to the front row in the classroom. Many children with spina bifida and hydrocephalus have problems with vision, and it is important that they should have the correct glasses prescribed and *wear* them.

Although crossed eyes are usually due to an imbalance of the eye muscles from birth (which causes double vision), some crossed eyes are due to another existing defect in vision. If a child has long or short sight, he will have to turn one eye in to focus properly and so he will appear to squint. This sort of squint is usually treated by glasses rather than surgery.

Many children intensely dislike wearing glasses; they are also inclined to drop and break them. It may be worth investing in non-breakable lenses for a wheelchair child, to reduce the risk of breakages if the glasses are allowed to fall on the floor. Conversely girls may be persuaded to take better care of their glasses by being allowed to choose a "fashion" style which appeals to their vanity as much as it improves their sight.

Children who are severely multiply handicapped and are profoundly deaf or totally or nearly blind will need very specialized services. There are many local groups with which national organizations are in touch and to which they can refer parents.

Going to the Dentist

Dental health is an integral part of our overall well-being and, unlike many other diseases, dental decay and gum disorders can be prevented throughout life with care and attention. One study in England and Wales found that 72 percent of handicapped children treated needed dental attention, compared with 32 percent of normal children. This survey found that mentally or multiply handicapped children, in particular, were likely to receive treatment only in an emergency. This would usually mean extraction, often with a general anesthetic.

Dental problems arise in children from a variety of causes, not the least our taste for candy, soft drinks, and the increasing number of medicines administered in syrup form. Handicapped children do not, of course, automatically suffer from increased dental problems and tooth decay compared with other children. But they currently appear to be more at risk. The reasons for this lack of treatment and cause of decay are various. Some children with, for example, cerebral palsy, may have deformities of the jaw which complicate dentistry and create irregular teeth. Cleaning may be difficult if the child cannot easily open his mouth or makes a wide range of sudden movements. Children with hemophilia or other bleeding problems will require inpatient treatment for extractions or major dental work, and other children with rheumatic or heart complaints may be at risk of infection after extractions. But these difficulties do not preclude treatment, and they are a powerful argument for regular checks and early attention to any problems.

Some handicapped children miss out on dental treatment simply because they attend residential institutions or special schools where there are limited facilities, and from which it is difficult for parents to fetch them for dental checks. An increasing number of schools for the physically handicapped are visited by mobile dental clinics, or provide transport to dentists at local centers. But a severely handicapped child who spends most of his time at home, or a handicapped child in a normal school, may not share these facilities. Some parents are additionally so overwhelmed by the logistics of caring for a handicapped child's everyday needs that they postpone the dentist's visit as a low priority. Others may hesitate to inflict on a handicapped child what they see as yet another trip to yet another specialist. Some children, particularly physically handicapped adolescents, may simply never go to the dentist because they cannot get there in a wheelchair.

Some dentists are reluctant to accept handicapped children. This may be because of the child's behavioral problems, or irregular and involuntary movements which complicate treatment. And some children with hemophilia or heart conditions may present complications if major work is required. Also, unfortunately, many dentists' offices are so inaccessible—up steep stairs or above stores and offices—that it is exceedingly difficult to get an older wheelchair child up to the office.

Treatment, however, does not have to be provided through a private dentists's office. It can be arranged at clinics, through the school dental service, or in hospital dental departments.

If parents have problems in finding a dentist willing to treat a handicapped child, community health councils can often help. Their knowledge of local services and their contacts in the community may produce a recommendation through the "grapevine." If not, they may take up the issue and try to establish a proper service. Older chronically sick and physically handicapped people have problems in common with children in finding dentists, and the issue is therefore much wider than parents might at first suppose. Many parents' groups have personal recommendations, and, if all else fails, the dental departments of hospitals (in particular teaching hospitals) are likely to be able to offer treatment.

Often physically handicapped children can be easily treated by their neighborhood dentist, if the parent explains in advance (and out of earshot of the child) what the problems are. The basis for acceptance or refusal is likely to be the child's degree of cooperation, and the extent of the physical handicap may bear no relation to tolerance in the dentist's chair. It is obviously desirable to establish working relationships with a *local* dentist, because of the convenience of access for checks and minor problems. The role of educator to the dentist may fall on the parent.

Apart from regular visits to the dentist, parents can play an important part in preventing trouble. Fluoride has proved its value in preventing trouble. Fluoride has proved its value in preventing dental decay in children, and fluoride tablets can be purchased from any druggist. The value of fluoride toothpastes and mouthwashes has been less clearly proven, but they may back up the work of the tablets. Although it has been suggested that toothpaste is useless, many children enjoy selecting and using their own brand. It is therefore worth purchasing this in order to make teeth cleaning a pleasurable process. Many children love electric toothbrushes, and where a child has poor hand control or finds it difficult to keep his mouth open and brush, these are likely to clean far more effectively. If brushing is impossible, teeth can still be cleaned with a piece of cloth wrapped around a finger.

Children with major brushing difficulties are likely to have major problems with decay—precisely because they are equally unlikely to be able to eat the crisp kinds of food which "self-clean" the teeth, and because they may well take a variety of medications which constantly coat the teeth with sticky substances. It is particularly important that candy is not used excessively as a "comforter" for the handicapped child. An early sweet tooth is likely to mean early tooth decay—although well-meaning family and friends certainly do not intend any discomfort to accompany their gifts of candy and chocolate. It is worth remembering, as a final thought, that some handicapped children will have enormous difficulty (because of the irregularity of their jaws and teeth) in having dentures fitted if they *do* lose their natural teeth. Equally, extraction may very well involve general anesthesia and possibly hospital admission. Therefore good teeth are essential for good health *and* personal convenience.

GENETIC COUNSELLING

Prevention of handicap by direct control of the causes is the ultimate aim of every progessive health service. With the increasing understanding of the genetic and other causes of handicapping conditions, there is a growing opportunity to avoid the ultimate disaster—the birth of a *second* handicapped child. If a family has had one handicapped child, parents should at once seek genetic counselling. In fact, they should receive this whether or not they intend to have further children. But such counselling is too often offered in an informal and inadequate manner. The advice to "go away and have another child" may be given, without real consideration of the risk of another damaged baby, and without taking full account of the emotional and personal vulnerability of the parents, and the possibility that they may have to face disturbing and hurtful decisions. Genetic counselling should be firmly based upon medical fact, where this is possible, and it should be given by specialists who are expert in this field.

The issue of prevention and health was brought to a head by the publication of a consultative document which indicates that, the diagnosis of disease in the fetus (unborn child) or in the mother is not new. Routine blood tests for pregnant women were introduced in the 1930s to diagnose syphilis; and tests for rhesus incompatability came in during the 1940s. These tests were, however, preludes to *treatment* which would offer a reasonable guarantee of producing a normal healthy child. During the 1960s and 1970s, techniques have been developed which enable geneticists and obstetricians to predict that a child will either suffer from a serious handicap or malformation, or that the mother is likely to have a child who will be handicapped.

These tests pose serious moral dilemmas. If parents know that their children might be handicapped, should they in fact have children at all? Certain handicapping conditions, like hemophilia and muscular dystrophy, are sex-linked disorders. In the Duchenne type of muscular dystrophy and hemophilia, the woman "carries" the abnormal gene, but only her male children are affected. If a woman carrier has a boy child, that child runs a fifty-fifty chance of being affected. If she has a girl child, that girl will not be affected. But she has a fifty-fifty chance of being a carrier, and her male children, in turn, may be handicapped. If parents are willing to take the risk of having a girl child, who might be a carrier, but not a boy, who would be affected, they can have a test called *amniocentesis*. A small sample of the amniotic fluid, which surrounds the baby in the womb, is withdrawn through a fine needle. This fluid is tested, and the sex of the child determined. If the parents have agreed to the test being carried out, they will normally abide by its conclusions. If the fetus is male, the pregnancy is terminated. If female, it is allowed to continue. Clearly, it is a difficult and unhappy decision for the family. But knowing the implications of hemophilia or muscular dystrophy from other family members, they may feel it to be the only humane and wise decision. Unfortunately, there is as yet no way of identifying whether the child has one of these two conditions in the fetus— only the sex of the child. Hence it is also possible that a boy might have been normal and unaffected. But many families would feel that this was an unwarrantable risk in view of the possible suffering and trauma.

Other handicapping conditions cannot be predicted from family history with any certainty. The precise cause of malformations of the central nervous system, which produce hydrocephalus, spina bifida, or anencephaly, are not known. However, a simple blood test has now been developed, which can be routinely carried out on all pregnant women. This is designed to gauge the level of alpha-proteins in the mother's blood. If the level is abnormally high, amniocentesis will be carried out. If this confirms an abnormally high level, termination can be performed. The abnormal protein levels appear to offer unequivocal proof of abnormality in the growing baby. The test is a sensitive one, and it is possible that the less severe forms of spina bifida might not be picked up. But it is a simple and very safe procedure to follow where there appears to be a reasonable risk of a damaged child.

Prenatal diagnosis is still in its infancy, and at present the only "treatment" for the diagnosis of an abnormal child is termination of pregnancy. Genetic counselling *before* pregnancy is confirmed would avoid the termination dilemma for those parents who were ethically opposed to it. It is very unlikely that any parents seeking termination of pregnancy would have difficulty in obtaining this through their local health service. However, as *Prevention and Health: Everybody's Business* (U. K. Department of Health and Social Security, 1976) comments, "prenatal diagnosis is a major technical advance which will become increasingly important in future but it poses ethical issues of great difficulty. It is society as a whole and not simply Government or the health professions alone that will have to try to resolve these questions." Until the financial implications of widespread screening, and the ethical issues involved in providing selective termination of pregnancy are resolved, the parents themselves will have to obtain the best advice possible and act accordingly ... bearing in mind that prevention is better than no cure.

5

Mobility Aids
Other Than Wheelchairs

GETTING AROUND
WITH THE VERY YOUNG CHILD

Very young handicapped children can travel around using the same equipment as their able-bodied brothers and sisters. However, they are likely to remain in need of these pieces of equipment well after other children of the same age are fully mobile, and their parents may need advice on the safest and most appropriate model of push-chair or stroller. Most young children now ride in baby buggies. These are lightweight folding pushchairs, with tubular metal frames and striped fabric hammock-type seats. Alvema Rehab's (Ortho-Kinetics, Inc.), "Minimax" or J. A. Preston Corporation's "Main-streamer Chair" are designed for larger and heavier disabled children. The "Twins Minimax" can also be purchased. The twin size is parti-

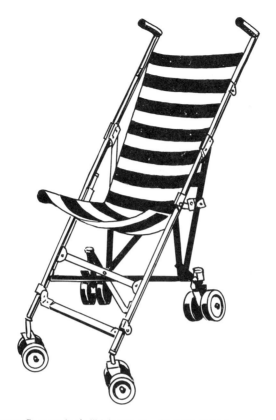

The J. A. Preston Corporation's "Mainstreamer Chair" is light to push and easy to fold.

cularly useful if a handicapped child and younger sibling have to be transported.

There is a wide range of strollers on the market, but many are very lightweight and small, to cater to the increasing need for collapsible models that can travel easily in cars and be conveniently dismantled for storage in small apartments and houses. Some of these strollers are not stable for larger children, and care should be taken in their selection if a child is likely to continue to use one after fifteen months.

There is a wide range of commercially produced slings, baby seats, and backpacks for carrying a small child and leaving the parents' hands free. These can be very useful if there are other small children in a family and it is necessary to travel on public transportation, or if a small child is fretful and unwilling to be left on his own. Small babies, in particular, enjoy close contact with their mothers and often sleep well in a sling-type carrier.

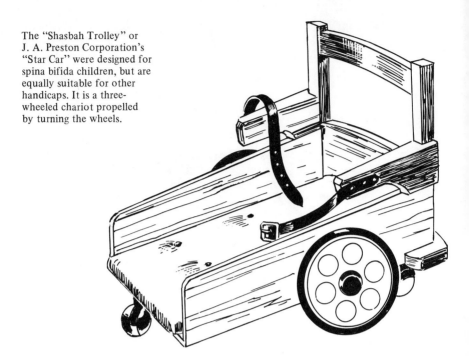

The "Shasbah Trolley" or
J. A. Preston Corporation's
"Star Car" were designed for
spina bifida children, but are
equally suitable for other
handicaps. It is a three-
wheeled chariot propelled
by turning the wheels.

Very few of the carriers, however, are suitable for a toddler with poor head control, and care should be taken with a child with spasms, since jerking forward can be dangerous in kitchen or bathroom areas where there are hard surfaces and the risk of scalds or burns.

As with other pieces of equipment designed to help a child pass from dependent to independent mobility, no one piece of equipment can suit every child, and parents need to assess suitability as they go on. The advantage of using equipment from standard ranges is that they can often be borrowed from neighbors or friends for a "trial run" to establish their suitability.

CANES AND CRUTCHES

Some children are eventually able to get out of their wheelchairs and walk limited distances with the aid of crutches or canes. Not all children will acquire skill with crutches, and many will never be able to master uneven ground, curbs, or stairs. But crutches are a useful adjunct to a wheelchair when moving in confined space, and they greatly facilitate entrance to public buildings when a wheelchair would be prohibitively large and cumbersome.

Underarm (axillary) crutches impose considerable strain on upper arms and shoulders, but offer good support if this is feasible. Elbow crutches have an armpiece to take weight above the elbow, and a handgrip. Forearm, trough, or gutter crutches are the most suitable for children with weak arm and hand control. The forearm rests in a paddy trough or gulley, with the hand gripping the handle or grip at the end of the trough.

The selection of an appropriate type of crutch should be fully discussed with the physical therapist. Children's crutches are normally adjustable, so that weight is properly distributed.

But whichever type is used, certain safety precautions should be observed. When using crutches, the child should try to adopt an upright posture, with head and shoulders in a natural position. If crutches are too short, they are dangerous because of the temptation to lean forward. Managing doors, stairs, sitting, and standing require practice. But wheelchairs can be adapted to carry crutches, and they will greatly extend a child's access to social activities and possibly work.

The extent to which a child uses his crutches depends upon the physical therapist's estimate of his skill. If he feels confident, he is probably all right. But some children (particularly with conditions like brittle bones where falls are hazardous) will never feel fully confident in crowded streets or school corridors. So if such a child attends a normal school, where corridors and playgrounds are busy and hazardous, it may be prudent to decide to use a wheelchair more than is strictly necessary to avoid accidents.

An important safety factor is the state of the ferrule, or rubber tip of the crutch. These tips should be kept in good condition, to make sure that there is no danger of slipping. Care should also be taken to ensure that the hand-grip covers are in good condition to avoid any unnecessary blistering or callouses. Children may get very hot and perspire more than usual when using axillary (underarm) crutches. In summer weather, natural fiber tee shirts or other absorbent play clothes may be practical and should be changed frequently.

A walking stick is the simplest form of mobility aid. Provided that there is adequate strength in the forearm and upper arm, it can be useful to wheelchair children as a pivot, or for partial weight-bearing when transferring from chair to bed, for instance. The conventional walking cane is probably of limited use to any wheelchair user, but a variety of adjustable sticks are available with quadruped bases. A quad cane is a four-legged tubular walking stick, with a variety of handles. Gutter or trough-type handles are interchangeable with crutches in some models, and offer a good deal of stability when balance is poor. To be safe and useful, sticks, like crutches, must be the correct height. The majority of children's sticks are fully adjustable, and a physical therapist will be able to advise on their proper use.

WALKERS

Walkers offer more elaborate support than canes. They fall into two basic types. One is light, usually made of tubular metal with rubber-tipped feet. This is basically for support and offers a stable base for standing. The second variety is intended to be pushed, rather than lifted, and sometimes is supplied with castor wheels. Care should be taken in the selection of a mobile type of frame, since some handicapped people feel very insecure if the frame appears to "run away" with them. Invacare's wheeled walker with braces overcomes this problem.

If space is at a premium, a child may find a dining chair on castors a convenient mobility aid. Smaller children can use the wide range of commercially produced pushing toys, provided that they are suitably weighted. If hard objects are used as ballast, they should be covered with thick cloth or suitable covering to avoid accident if the child falls on top of them.

Very handicapped or very young children may need walking frames similar to the baby walkers available for able bodied children from eighteen months and older. Infant and toddler training walkers

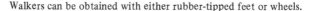

Walkers can be obtained with either rubber-tipped feet or wheels.

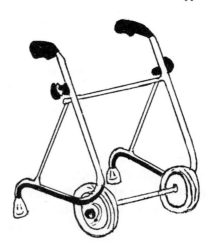

and cerebral palsy walkers with padded balance rings are available from Invacare. Children's walkers with overhead frames are also available.

No mobility aid will achieve its object if the room in which it is used is cluttered with toys, furniture, loose rugs, and electric cords. If possible, it is preferable to arrange furniture to give maximum floor space and to rule out any risk of damage through bumps and scratches.

BRACES

Some wheelchair children will be able to walk for varying distances with splints or braces. The type of brace that a child needs will depend upon the experience and professional opinion of the hospital consultant and physical therapist. Many small children will start with long, full-length braces with abdominal and chest bands. These full-length braces are fitted when there is damage high in the spine and the body muscles are paralyzed or inadequate from the site of the defect downward. Since the point of wearing braces is to remedy muscular defects which prevent the joint from functioning properly, some children will improve and may progress to full-length leg braces with ring or bucket tops or even to short below-the-knee braces. The progress may be slow and gradual, and braces should always be worn and treated specifically according to instructions.

The design of conventional braces does not appear to have changed since the 1930s, but cosmetic braces are now available. While these are not perhaps necessary for younger children, they will improve the morale of an adolescent girl who is extremely conscious of her disability.

Two young girls in an English survey, who were both polio victims, obtained cosmetic braces, but both had trouble with them. The footpieces were too large, with the result that they could not get proper shoes to combine with the brace. One girl could not get to the shoe store because she had no other brace. The other was unwilling to go into the shop wearing her old brace, take it off in public, and put on the new one to try shoes. In fact, the braces were neither efficient nor cosmetic (since efficiency and good design are closely linked), and there was a clear impression that the designs had not been followed closely enough.

These two cases illustrate the problems caused by separation of fitting and manufacturing. They additionally indicate that parents need to be alert to the possibility of better fitting or better designed braces, if they feel that they are not receiving a proper service. In the majority of cases, the doctor issuing the original prescription will not be present at the final fitting and handing over of an appliance. It may be helpful to ask that a physical therapist or occupational therapist should make a last check to see that the appliance will carry out the function intended and that it fits. Patients who appreciated their consultant's or doctor's interest and attention, nevertheless regretted the lack of firm medical direction in seeing that the appliances prescribed really met the needs of a disability. It is clearly essential that each appliance should be checked on delivery by someone in the hospital who can assess that it will be satisfactory. Many disabled people believe that services will not improve until technicians are attached to *individual* hospitals, so that alterations and repairs can be carried out more simply.

Any parent acquiring braces should enquire about repairs at the time. Despite their tough appearance, braces can break. Families do not automatically receive repair braces, and they should not be worn when screws are lost, straps broken or frayed or stitching insecure. Children grow, and in view of the time lag between ordering and delivery, they may have grown in size by delivery, and they are in any case more likely than adults to expose their braces to active and rough play. It would seem very sad for an eight-year-old child to be prohibited from football and other playground games played with crutches and braces because he might render himself totally wheelchair bound by breaking a brace.

When suitable braces have been obtained, they need to be used correctly. Very young childen will receive help from the physical therapist in standing and walking practice. It may be possible to borrow parallel bars to assist with any exercises the hospital recommends. Because braces can cause great problems if they rub or cease to fit adequately, attention should always be paid to the child's skin. Reddening or bruising means that the device is incorrectly adjusted, or that the fit is wrong. Braces can be hot, and the limbs affected should be washed carefully with soap and water each night. If the child has very sensitive skin, tights may be more comfortable under the appliance, then socks and trousers over it. Another cause of injury is, again, the inability of the paraplegic or spina bifida child to feel sensation below the waist, so special care should be taken with hot radiators or sharp toys while the child is moving around.

It should perhaps be stressed that there is currently a good deal of experimentation in the design of braces, particularly for use by severely handicapped children in their early days of walking. These experimental braces are available only through individual hospitals, and represent the particular philosophy and treatment recommended by an individual consultant. Overenthusiastic use is as bad as underuse. Many older children, on the other hand, may choose to concentrate on their wheelchairs rather than crutches, braces, or walking aids. This may be a realistic choice in the long term, but it is vital for physical development that all children should have at least a chance to walk and stand.

Many parents feel very disturbed when they first see a child trying to get along in braces. He may appear very clumsy and disoriented, and they are nervous of bumps and falls. However, most children will find even minimal walking skills very rewarding and will improve with practice. Additionally any exercise will strengthen muscles and bones and reduce the risk of fractures in the long run. Some children will need canes and/or crutches in addition to braces, and the physical therapist may be able to suggest exercises for strengthening the arm and shoulder muscles. There are a number of games that involve stretching and pulling, and that encourage balance and confidence.

What each child needs to succeed is encouragement to go on trying. If a child suspects that his mother secretly wishes that he would stay safely in the wheelchair, because of the time spent in adjusting braces or because of his own tumbles around the house, he may simply give in and cease to try. If parents feel that braces are not achieving any results, they should ask their physical therapist and ensure that they fully understand fitting and use. Some of the braces used for spina bifida children, for example, have pelvic and chest bands and straps to control the hips. Very often these full-length braces will be replaced by ring-top or braces that are below the knee, but progress will only be ensured if parents persist and follow advice implicitly.

Children using walking appliances should be dressed suitably. If knee joints rub trouser legs or skirts, they can be padded with soft leather. Skirts, if long, can act as camouflage. But they should not be so long that the child can catch a heel and fall.

OTHER MOBILITY AIDS

Young handicapped children have exactly the same need to explore their environment as their able-bodied brothers and sisters. Since a wheelchair is scarcely a flexible tool with which to sample the feel of the kitchen floor, the movement of a door hinge, or the hidden world under the table, something has to be found to substitute for natural movement.

Crawling aids can be purchased, which offer a support for the chest, usually mounted on a tubing frame with castor wheels. Invacare's "Crawler" is one commercially manufactured crawler that can be adjusted to the child's arms and chest, but it is possible to manufacture simple models for home use with padded wooden frames and castor wheels. Some children can also use the range of crawling toys which are on the market for normal children. A crawler is also useful for playing at floor level, since with it the child has far greater mobility and reach than on a foam wedge or beanbag. As it is important that the child learns to propel himself along in a way that will not impede future development or encourage bad posture, the physical therapist's advice should be sought about the most appropriate equipment.

Perhaps the most difficult mobility aid to find is a suitable mobility toy. There are a number of baby walkers for pushing or walking (on frames) on the open market; but by the time a handicapped child is sufficiently developed to use them, they are likely to prove too small or short. Additionally some handicapped children put more weight and stress on one part of a piece of equipment than able-bodied children, and they tend to have minor accidents as a result. But many normal baby walkers or trucks may be quite suitable for a handicapped child if they are suitably weighted to prevent them from "running away" (see page 100). All young children love trucks, and the baby walker is a great incentive to mobility.

Some very young children benefit from the use of a "baby bouncer," which is available from most children's shops and which can be suspended from a door frame or individual stand. Baby bouncers are excellent for stimulating leg movements, but great care should be taken not to let a handicapped child use them for too long. There is some medical evidence which suggests that excessive use (arising, for instance, if the child falls asleep while swinging) can cause poor posture and reinforce any muscular abnormalities. Small children should *never* be allowed to slump in the bouncer, and it should be used for very short periods. Care should also be taken to ensure that the canvas sling is properly adjusted and that the back muscles are supported. The same care should be taken with any mobility equipment (also particularly with the baby walker) to prevent the child from becoming tired and sinking into uncomfortable and awkward positions. The purpose of activity equipment is to teach and reinforce physical activity; but misuse can have the reverse—and extremely damaging—effect.

Some children like toys which they can sit astride and push along with a little use of their legs. Again, there are a range of small horses, cars, and trains on the market (usually made of plastic) which may be suitable.

A number of aids are available for sitting and steering. The "Shasbah Trolley" was designed for spina bifida children, but is equally suitable for others. The trolley is a three-wheeled chariot propelled by turning the wheels. Because it is so low, there is little chance of even a very small child falling, and many children learn to use it very skillfully. The majority of children find them enjoyable both indoors and in the garden, and they are usually very popular with able-bodied friends and siblings. An alternative to the trolley is the J. A. Preston Corporation's "Whizz." This is hand-operated and is propelled and steered by moving the handle. The "Whizz" is suitable for four- to nine-year-olds who sit in the molded plastic frame.

For children who are unable to pedal a standard tricycle, hand-propelled tricycles are now available in this country. Strictly speaking they are not tricycles in the conventional sense of the word, but resemble go-carts. The "Irish Mail" is also hand-operated. It moves when the handle is pumped back and forth. It is suitable for indoor use.

A lot of children gain pleasure from riding a tricycle—which is a much more "normal" mobility aid than a wheelchair. Since most children who need a wheelchair will be unable to operate the conventional foot pedal mechanism, it will be necessary to purchase a modified tricycle or adapt an existing model.

There is an increasingly strong and attractive range of mobility toys available in the stores, and it may be possible to purchase a standard pedal or battery car and modify this slightly for use by a handicapped child. Any wheelchair child will get good value from a mobility toy which is safe, suitable, and "normal" looking. so it may be worth borrowing neighbor's toys to assess their value. Most manufacturers are now sympathetic to the needs of handicapped children and will advise on stability and durability; they will often provide or make practical suggestions on any minor modifications required. Some hospitals and social services departments can lend or provide mobility toys, and the physical therapist's opinion and experience are invaluable. In the end, choice naturally depends upon the degree

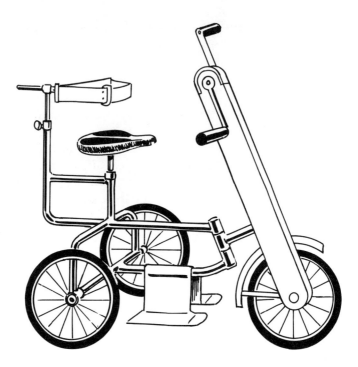

Hand-propelled tricycles are popular with children between four and ten years of age. Most can be ridden in braces and have a range of foot and back rests.

of handicap and the resulting physical ability. However, many handicapped children underfunction (especially when young) because they lack appropriate stimulation or the opportunity to learn new physical skills. Very often the provision of a very basic piece of play equipment like the tire on wheels produces improvement through experimentation and effort. Care should be taken, however, that toys bought on the open market do not reinforce the child's handicap by encouraging abnormal posture, and that they are strong enough to take the sometimes considerable extra stress which a handicapped child may put on a mobility toy.

TRAVEL BY CAR

Cars are vital for wheelchair families. As one mother put it, "the car is the family's legs." Although very young physically handicapped children can be taken on public transport using baby buggies, the difficulty of lifting an immobile child of four or five, shopping basket, and pushchair all together has to be experienced to be believed.

When a child is too heavy to take on public transport, the alternative is often walking. In bad or cold weather, the family may become virtually immobile unless a family friend or relative can help.

If a car is available, there are a variety of ways of making journeys convenient and easy. A small child will not present a majo problem in getting in the car, since he can be transferred directly from the wheelchair to a car seat. Car seats or safety harnesses are essential for all handicapped children, since physical handicap frequently impairs the sense of balance. If a handicapped child rolls with the movement of the car, he may not be able spontaneously to recover his balance, and can fall and catch head or hands on door handles. Additionally, harnesses and car seats offer support to weak backs and necks. There are a number of car seats on the market which are suitable for all children; selection should be based on individual choice. Car seats should be carefully fitted in accordance with the manufacturer's instructions. If in doubt, a garage should be consulted for advice. A useful harness requiring no fixed anchor points and more support and security than the conventional seat belt is available.

Comfort is important for a handicapped person, who may find the position he has to adopt in a car tiring or painful. Sheepskin seat covers offer protection from pressure sores and prevent the perspiration that can be caused by plastic car seat covers in conjunction with braces or plastic incontinence clothes. Special backrests or headrests can be purchased from car accessory shops. If a paraplegic or cerebral palsy traveler has muscle spasms, it may be necessary to maintain the limbs in a suitable position with foam or polystyrene-filled cushions. Handicapped children, like any children, will also get bored on long journeys, and a sensible collection of small toys and ideas for games should be provided.

Getting into the Car

If a child is heavy and cannot transfer directly from his wheelchair, a travel seat is useful. This is a two-handled carrying seat which can be lifted out of the wheelchair directly into the car. Travel seats are also useful for carrying into theaters, restaurants, or restricted areas where a wheelchair is unusable. They are safest if carried by two people. If stairs are involved in access to a car (as in a basement garage in an apartment building) it may be preferable to carry the wheelchair folded and use the travel seat or an ambulance chair. Ambulance chairs are lightweight rigid chairs with canvas seats. They have back wheels for pushing and are useful for carrying children with poor back and head control. Two people are needed for lifting.

If direct transfer to the car from a wheelchair is required, and it is not possible to use crutches, a walker frame, or a cane, the wheelchair should be maneuvered until it is adjacent to the seat. The arm rest on the side of the seat should be removed, and a child with strong arms should be able to slide directly onto the car seat. Some disabled people find a transfer board is essential as a bridge between the chair and car seat, particularly if the car seat is rather lower than the seat of the wheelchair. Transfer boards can be purchased or made. They are usually made of highly polished wood (which must be regularly checked for splinters or roughness). It will be much easier to get into a two-door than a four-door car, because of the additional space. If sliding is impractical, a handgrip fixed to the car roof may help the child to swing in from the chair. It is sometimes easier to get into a car seat backward, and lift the legs around and in afterward. Rotating car seats can be purchased. These seats, which can be fitted to any car, swing around and out beyond the doorway, removing the necessity to maneuver the handicapped person out of the chair and into a fixed seat within the confines of the car. There are also a number of car lifts available (like the Hoyer chrome travel lifter [Everest and Jennings, Inc.]). These lifts are attached to the roof of the car and swing the passenger into the car seated on a sling. Alternatively a mobile lift can be used, similar to those recommended in Chapter 6 for bedroom and bathroom use. All lift and sling equipment needs care and attention in use and maintenance, and many parents may feel it is not worth the bother. But it is worth looking to the future when things may not seem so simple—and when the small child may be a very heavy teenager. Manufacturers are usually willing to arrange home demonstrations, and it cannot be stressed sufficiently that any complex aid of this nature must be demonstrated and used first under observation to avoid danger and ensure minimum inconvenience.

Motorized Transport
for Severely Handicapped Children

If families find it convenient to transport a severely handicapped older child in his wheelchair traveling, vans and minibuses can be converted to carry disabled people. Ford vans and, Chrysler and Volkswagen minibuses and vans can be modified through arrangement with dealers. Quotations will usually be made for individual modifications, and it is important that the correct specifications are given. Because adaptations are skilled, it may be difficult to find a manufacturer willing to undertake adaptations on a secondhand vehicle. An exception is the conversion of minivans. These vans can be converted so that the roof is raised, with additional windows, to encompass the height of wheelchair and passenger. A folding ramp comes down from the rear of the van for entrance and exit. Some system of fork-lift platform is usually required on the larger and higher vans. They are powered by an electrohydraulic unit connected to the vehicle battery and are usually essential on all cars.

If wheelchairs are transported with passengers in a vehicle, it is absolutely essential that safety precautions are enforced. Wheelchairs must have their brakes on and should be clamped to the floor of the vehicle. L. Mulholland Corporation makes tie downs that ensure that the chair cannot move. Certain wheelchairs are difficult to secure, and advice should be sought from the manufacturers before fitting clamps. Wheelchairs can be immobilized in transit by webbing straps (similar to seatbelts), and if the floor fittings are secure, this method is usually cheaper and simpler to operate. Since straps can pull out if improperly adjusted, thought should also be given to the user before adopting a particular system. The clamp system will usually take the most weight and most completely immobilize the chair. If a chair moves forward and falls (on a bend or in an accident), the child restrained in the chair will also fall forward with the full weight of the chair on top of him.

Learning to Drive

An adolescent may manage to drive his parents' car; if this skill is combined with competent management of the wheelchair, it will give him a considerable degree of personal freedom. Cars with automatic transmission will almost always be easiest for a disabled person to manage. A number of firms will adapt a car so that a disabled person can drive it. Demonstrations and trial drives can be arranged to test the various hand-operated or foot-operated controls. It is quite possible to drive a converted car with one hand or one leg, and hand-operated cars can also be hired from Avis Rent-a-Car.

Most adolescents are anxious to drive, but parents should of course assess their overall maturity and competence, as well as their physical capability. Driving in heavy traffic is stressful and difficult, and a very sheltered child may need more than average instruction in basic road sense and safety precautions.

The advantage in having an adapted family car is that outings can be social occasions. The motorized three-wheeler has met mobility needs for many individuals, but it is very cramped for wheelchair transport and cannot carry passengers. It also has been criticized severely for basic design faults which have included susceptibility to cross winds, mechanical failures, and poor road-holding properties.

TRAVEL BY BUS

The older physically handicapped child, with a larger wheelchair, is unlikely to be able to travel on a bus. A younger child, who can travel in a baby buggy or pushchair may be eligible for a free bus pass because of his disability. Many bus companies do not charge for children under the age of five years, whether handicapped or able-bodied, and the concession is most likely to be relevant to the five-to nine-year-old group. Some buses now have special seats for the disabled or elderly and (provided that there is suitable space for the chair) may give additional mobility to families without a car or living some distance from stores and shopping centers.

TRAVEL BY AIR

Airlines are usually well equipped to meet the needs of the wheel-chair traveler. It is, however, absolutely essential to give ample advance notification of any special requirements and a statement that the child will be traveling with a wheelchair.

Most airports will remove the wheelchair upon checking in and process it with the rest of the luggage. An airport wheelchair will normally be provided to cover the waiting period and transfer to the plane. Facilities for actually getting a wheelchair passenger on and off planes vary greatly according to the airport. For children who are not too heavy and have some mobility, a travel seat or other carrier may be preferred. Some airlines will permit a baby buggy to be regarded as cabin luggage so that it may be taken directly onto the plane; but this is discretionary and may depend upon the passenger load on a particular flight.

Some airlines, for technical reasons, treat a disabled person as one who is sick and may require a medical certificate. If any special attention is required on the flight, or if a certificate is likely to be requested, it is prudent to book a few weeks before flying in order to iron out any questions or problems.

Since aircraft have little walking space and seats are close together, it will probably be impossible to maneuver inside the aircraft with any walking aid. Therefore, the handicapped person will need assistance and support from a parent in going to the toilet. An important point to remember for unaccompanied children is that stewardesses and hostesses are not allowed to help passengers in the bathrooms. This ruling relates to hygiene requirements regarding serving of food in the air, but it means that some handicapped people will not be able to get to the toilet on an unaccompanied flight without the goodwill of a fellow passenger. This may be a major problem.

It is also wise to check arrangements at the airport in the city or country of arrival, to make certain that provision is made for access to customs and reunion with the wheelchair. Small airports in holiday resorts may lack many of the facilities of international airports. However, goodwill will usually provide alternatives if reasonable notice is given.

TRAVEL BY BOAT

Ferries and cruise ships contain many hazards to the able-bodied —steep stairs, inaccessible bathrooms, and multistoried facilities. However, most ships have elevators and the crew will make alternative arrangements if requested in advance. Generally speaking, large boats are not suitable for vacations for people in wheelchairs, because of the problems of levels, but in combination with a car they may be a more convenient method of transport than air travel.

6

Choosing and Using
a Wheelchair

OBTAINING A WHEELCHAIR

Usually the doctor concerned will recommend a particular model of chair and the appliance center where it is available, with the proposal that the child should visit the center and be measured and assessed for a chair by a technician. It will be possible to try a number of chairs at the center, and it is important that parents attend the center with the child. If a chair is to be pushed as well as self-propelled, it is necessary that modifications are suited to the attendant *and* occupant. Some appliance centers will send a technician to the child's home to assess the home environment and make recommendations taking these into account. Since a wheelchair is intended to be a pair of legs rather than a comfortable armchair (though the best wheelchairs will combine the two distinct functions quite well), it is very

112

important to pick a model that will negotiate narrow corridors or awkward corners without too much difficulty; that can be pushed up or down any small steps or ramps without problems; and that the child can use for access to the bathroom and all family amenities to the best of his ability. Wheelchair clinics will often be able to send a physical therapist or occupational therapist for a home assessment and parents should request such a visit if they feel it would be useful.

Electric wheelchairs may also be purchased through an appliance center. But although a doctor may recommend a particular model, the appliance center will take the major step in deciding which type of electrically powered wheelchair (if any) is suitable for an individual applicant.

Because of the problems involved in providing a chair that meets the precise specifications for individual disabled people, an increasing number of hospitals how have special wheelchair clinics to provide assessment and practical guidance for children and adults. When it is possible, therefore, to attend a wheelchair clinic, it is clearly in the interests of the child to do so. The wheelchair clinic will ensure access to physical therapists and occupational therapists, in addition to hospital consultants who are expert in the particular problems of an individual disability. In many cases, appliance centers are acting on the instructions of an absent doctor, who may or may not have taken into account the particular problems of selecting a wheelchair to meet the combined needs of good postural support, maximum individual mobility, suitability to the family home, and maneuverability by parents. The family doctor's problems in making recommendations are clear, and the wheelchair clinic can ensure that the appropriate chair is chosen and that (most importantly) it takes future growth into account. A severely handicapped child may be further handicapped by the use of an unsuitable chair that aggravates his deformities and encourages bad posture. If a wheelchair prescription is made with insufficient knowledge of the range of chairs and the child's physical and environmental needs, the result is clearly going to be unsatisfactory. Additionally it is not the role of an appliance center to teach a child how to use a wheelchair (although visitors to a center will have an opportunity to try chairs). Wheelchair clinics however can provide training programs both in general mobility and safety requirements, and also in transfers from chair to bath, toilet, or bed. If a child is severely handicapped and totally dependent upon family help, parents will also need instruction for their appropriate posture in using the chair and in lifting—both for their own backs and for the prevention of future deformities in the child.

THE BASIC REQUIREMENTS
OF A WHEELCHAIR

Although parents may often feel inadequate and incompetent in the face of the special needs of their handicapped child—and bewildered by the confusing choices which seem to face them when considering wheelchairs and other appliances—they can help themselves and their child by having some idea of what they are looking for in a chair. The energetic paraplegic boy with strong arm and chest muscles may look for a lightweight and tough wheelchair, with high maneuverability, in order to enjoy wheelchair sports and to achieve a great degree of personal independence. A very young child may need a chair with a tray and which is easily pushed. If a child is going to use either a powered or self-propelled chair independently outside the house, it is important to see that the braking system is both strong and accessible. For a severely handicapped child (in particular one with cerebral palsy where all four limbs may be severely affected), a special chair may be required which can tip to alter the sitting position, can offer special foot supports to compensate for spasms, and perhaps alternative sets of road and indoor wheels so that the chair is usable inside and outside the house. Some families, particularly in rural areas, may be heavily dependent upon car or public transport, and a lightweight folding model may be essential. Additionally, the accessories available for particular models vary. The school child may need removable arm rests in order to sit normally at a desk or table. Because wheelchairs vary between providing an occasional outing and offering the sole means of independent mobility—and because houses and apartments have very different space and storage facilities—any decision should be based on a balanced professional and personal decision.

THE MAIN TYPES OF WHEELCHAIRS

Self-Propelled Wheelchairs

Self-propelled wheelchairs are moved by pushing the large wheels with the hands. They can also be pushed by an attendant using the handles. Self-propelled chairs are intended to act as genuine independence aids, and they must therefore be chosen to fit in with the home environment. Most adult self-propelled chairs vary in width between 22 and 26 in. (560 to 660 mm). As many doors are only

24 in. wide (610 mm), particularly to bathrooms or in awkward corridor turns, it is sensible to choose a chair as narrow as is comfortable. The width selected should allow for clothing and any cushions or pads on the chair seat. Self-propelled wheelchairs are usually moved by hand operation of the back wheels. In cases where a child has poor shoulder control, it is possible on some models to have the action reversed and the large wheels placed at the front of the wheelchair. Large front wheels, however, make it difficult to transfer sideways into bed or onto the commode, and they are awkward for attendants to push. Because the weight of the large wheel is on the front of the chair, it is not possible to tip the chair to mount curbs or minor obstacles, and personal movement is therefore diminished. Sometimes the problem of weak shoulder or hand control can be overcome by the fitting of *capstans*, or inner rings, to the wheels so that the hands can grip and turn more easily.

Most self-propelled chairs fold for transport, and it is possible to obtain extra lightweight chairs (weighing about 30 lb, compared with the usual 50 lb or more) if lifting is likely to be a problem. Lightweight chairs, obviously, are not as sturdy as the heavier models and are usually recommended only for the more delicate child who would have difficulty in propelling a heavier chair. They are not suitable for extensive outdoor use.

Small children will probably initially use a pushchair outside the house, rather than a wheelchair. One of the smallest self-propelled wheelchairs available is the "Martin 601," manufactured by Alvema Rehab. A "Travel Chair" manufactured by Ortho-Kinetics, Inc. is developed from the idea of a car seat. It has a seat width of 12 in. (340 mm) and a seat depth of 12 in. (340 mm). Its weight at 24 lbs. makes it very maneuverable, and it has adjusted footrests and a detachable tray.

Children plainly come in all sizes, and some children need larger chairs much earlier than others. Everest and Jennings' "Active Duty Light Weight" model is an alloyed metal all-purpose folding chair. It can be carried in most cars. Its weight at 32.5 lbs. (15.2 kg) makes the chair reasonable to carry, and a number of special design features can be incorporated, including detachable armrests for work at a table or desk, detachable footrests, and front rigging.

It is essential to note children's growth needs. Everest and Jennings sells a "growing" chair for children that adjusts with their progress. Chairs that are too large, however, may create postural deformities, especially if the child's legs do not hang naturally over the edge of the seat. Most chairs have adjusted footrests and backrests, and care should be taken that these are comfortable for supporting, not deforming, the child.

Attendant-Operated Chairs

Some children are quite unable to propel their own chairs and need to be pushed. The "Responder Chair" (available from Modular Medical Corp.) is a newly designed modular positioning and travel chair for the handicapped child. With a child in it, it will fit onto a seat in a car or in public transportation in minutes. It has retractable wheels that can be set in six different reclining positions. This is useful for the severely handicapped, since the chair can be tilted either for resting or change of position. The chair also has a footrest coated in vinyl and has medial-lateral channels for foot positioning. Alvema Rehab's "Max 303" is an outdoor pushchair with a seat width of 13.25 in. (335 mm). It can only carry children between the ages of five and ten, but can be supplied with a variety of accessories including a weatherproof raincape, pelvic harness, shoulder harness, leg rests, and headrest. A folding hood is also available for bad weather.

Spinal carriages are seldom required nowadays, since wheelchairs are available in more sophisticated models, and pushchairs have optional accessories such as leg rests. For those children and adults who have severe handicaps and are unable to maintain seated posture, Everest and Jennings offers the "Multi-Care Chair" and the "Multi-Position Chair." These chairs have castor wheels for easier rides, positioning straps, specially tapered seat cushions, and assorted bolsters for positioning. The "Multi-Care Chair" can be folded for storage and transportation.

Transit Chairs

Car transit chairs are useful for many families, particularly for limited movement around the house or for moving a heavy child out of the car. In the latter case, the wheelchair is kept folded in the car trunk or garage. Car transit chairs usually have either four 12-in. wheels, or two back 12-in. wheels and two front castors. Although they cannot be propelled with the hands, as in a conventional wheelchair, they can be "punted" along with one or two canes or with a cane and a foot. They are often not particularly easy to push, since the castors mean that the chair swivels easily, but they can be very useful on vacation or for movement where space is limited along a corridor to a bathroom. The Everest and Jennings' "Glideabout" is the smallest of these chairs, 20 in. wide (508 mm). With removable armrests (making sideways transfers easy), it is virtually a dining-room chair on wheels.

A number of different chairs for "paddling along" are available. Some families make their own glideabout chairs by mounting ordinary kitchen chairs on castors for use in living rooms or bedrooms. These chairs are clearly not suitable for the severely handicapped, but can make life simpler for the more able-bodied disabled. It is important, when adapting a chair for this type of use, to shorten the legs, so that the child's feet can touch the floor. If there is no movement in the feet, it may be easier to mount the whole chair on a small platform with castors underneath, and rely on a cane or hand movement on furniture or walls for propulsion.

Ambulance chairs can also be obtained for lifting disabled people in confined spaces. These chairs have to be carried by two people, and normally have lightweight tubular frames and canvas seats. They are convenient for mounting steep stairways or traveling between wheelchair and vehicle on journeys. The "Trans-Sit" seat, a drip-dry nylon seat with carrying handles fitted inside the wheelchair, can lift a disabled person easily and does not require any special skill from the two helpers. Because this seat folds down to a size of 4 in. by 18 in., it can be a useful extra on journeys or when visiting friends, dentists, hairdressers, and so forth when a wheelchair may not be welcome or have adequate access.

Electric Wheelchairs
in the Home

If a child can propel himself for limited distances, but has difficulty in managing for long without exhaustion (or if he needs a powered chair to participate in all the activities at school or in a center), an electric wheelchair will normally be best.

There are a wide range of privately manufactured electric-powered chairs on the market. Everest and Jennings' "Powerdrive" is a strong indoor chair which can be used to a limited extent outside the house. It is available in junior and adult models, and can be pushed by an attendant if the battery runs down or the chair breaks down. Some models, however, cannot be pushed or freewheeled. This is not so important if the chair is used only inside the house, but it can be desperately inconvenient if the chair stops at the end of a long sidewalk outside.

Electric powered wheelchairs can obviously have more sophisticated steering than self-propelled models. Some wheelchairs can have microcontrols fitted which require minimal arm movement. Some will be steered by a central or side column, (as with the Batricar, the model manufactured by Braune of Stroud (Batric). These central controls make some wheelchair users feel safer (since it would be very difficult to fall out of the chair), but they can make getting in and out of the chair more difficult. If a child is very severely handicapped, the steering can be power-assisted on many models, or can be adapted to respond to any residual ability (movements of the chin, fingers, or feet on the controls, or by a suck-blow mechanism). Steering controls can usually be mounted on either side of a chair, according to need. Manufacturers will indicate the capacity of a chair. Some, like the "Fireball Junior Chair," made by Biddle Engineering Co., Ltd. (BEC), have variable speeds in reverse and forward gears. Capacity without recharging the battery will vary with the model, the weight of the child, and the wheelchair. Manufacturers indicate probable expectations of mileage before recharge is necessary—generally outdoor chairs offer better mileage since they are heavier, larger, and can sometimes run on two batteries simultaneously to permit journeys of up to six miles to be made.

Parents often wonder at what age a young child can be given a powered chair. The final decision will obviously rest with the wheelchair clinic or appliance center, but in general a child would probably be of school age. It is, in any event, in a child's interests to learn to become self-sufficient if possible in a conventional wheelchair, a "Shasbah Trolley," or on the "Whizz 33" (manufactured by J. A. Preston Corporation) before acquiring a powered chair. Powered chairs break, like all other mechanical objects, and the child who cannot manage an alternative mobility aid will have considerable difficulty while waiting for his chair to be mended. If a powered chair is used all the time, arm and shoulder muscles will lose strength, and self-propulsion will be difficult. If at all possible, children should start with tricycles, wheelchairs, or trolleys and keep up these skills even after a more sophisticated powered mobility aid has been acquired. If a powered chair is needed for a small child, there are suitable chairs, such as the Bambino. This chair is built onto a solid wooden frame, with an upholstered seat. The control is similar to that on the popular adult BEC powered wheelchair, with a small joy stick mounted on one or other of the arm rests. The chair has larger front wheels, with pneumatic tires, and can therefore manage more pavement or outside use than indoor chairs with smaller wheels.

A number of special powered wheelchairs are available which are powered platforms rather than conventional wheelchairs. These chairs are basically office chairs on powered platforms. The advantage of chairs like the Chairmobile is primarily their adaptability in an office or work setting. Because of their height, users can face rather than look up to colleagues, and there is no restriction on the use of arms or upper body. The platform can be adjusted to carry a normal chair or stool (providing that its back legs are not more than 17.5 in. (440 mm) apart.

A powered chair can revolutionize a disabled child's life. Care should be taken, however, to make a selection on the basis of reason rather than random choice. Many families have storage problems, and a chair like the popular BEC models which fold easily once the battery has been unplugged and removed, are good choices. Depending on whether the rear or front wheels are motorized, a chair may be good or bad at mounting slopes or curbs, or at being pushed if the battery runs down. The home or school terrain may be an important factor in choosing between two chairs. Powered chairs are not cheap, and maintenance, batteries, and repairs may make them costly mobility aids. It is therefore absolutely essential to explore the market and seek professional advice. Consultants and physical therapists at rehabilitation centers or wheelchair clinics are usually well informed about the whole range of chairs on the market, and their advice (as well as that of manufacturers) should be sought.

Selecting a Wheelchair for Outside Use

Most handicapped people will sometimes wish to use a wheelchair outside the house. If this use is usually only transport to and from a car, the normal lightweight folding wheelchair used in the house will probably be quite adequate. But if small journeys are to be made on pavement or roads or if the yard is hilly and rough, a more substantial chair will be required. Electric-powered wheelchairs provide the most convenient form of outside access.

Outdoor wheelchairs do not have to have the same maneuverability as indoor chairs, where space may be at a premium. It is stability that is all important outside, particularly if the chair is to be used on steep gradients. Some wheelchairs can climb steep gradients and even pull small garden trolleys, although these resemble minitractors rather than conventional wheelchairs. Generally speaking, the indoor chair will need a short wheelbase, a fairly narrow track, and a good steering lock. This will make the chair easy to manipulate in narrow doorways or at turns in corridors. The outside wheelchair will need a long wheelbase, a wide track, and more limited steering, so as to be more stable because it is close to the ground and there is little risk of tipping.

Outdoor chairs need good brakes. Many chairs have handbrakes for additional safety. These are a sensible precaution, but a child with weak hand muscles may find them difficult to put on or off. It is therefore important to *try* a variety of models before selecting one for purchase.

Powered wheelchairs are much heavier than the conventional self-propelled wheelchairs, particularly if they are designed for outside and rough use. This means that if a chair breaks down, it may not be possible to push it because of the weight of the motor. Some chairs have motors which can be disconnected so that the chair can be pushed, but otherwise a van will have to be procured to get the chair home. Other chairs have a special position for the control stick which enables the chair to be free-wheeled by an attendant, so that the chair can be moved. Lifting a powered chair in and out of a van is hard work, unless there is a hydraulic lift, and it may be essential for some families to choose a chair which can be brought home on foot if there is a breakdown. An alternative is to find a friendly garage attendant who will come to the rescue in an emergency.

Powered chairs have a limited range, depending upon their motor and battery capacity. The range of a chair, before recharging of the battery is required, will vary from four to twelve miles. Some chairs have charges incorporated in the chair, which saves a good deal of difficulty. Enquiries about precise mileage to be expected should be made from manufacturers. Hilly districts will obviously put more strain on a motor than flat level areas, and the mileage may be reduced.

Batteries must be watched very carefully on outside chairs. They will normally require recharging every night, either by a separate unit (which must be obtained with the chair) or through their own built-in charging unit. When a battery begins to wear out, a powered chair may speed along on flat sidewalks, but stick when asked to climb more than very shallow gradients. If the chair is very heavy and it sticks at the bottom of a hill, there will be problems in getting it up. Attention should therefore be paid to wheelchair performance and the first signs of any battery inadequacy.

It is almost always easier to manage curbs and other obstacles in a self-propelled wheelchair than in a powered chair; the large wheels of the self-propelled chair make it easier to tip the chair slightly, and it is possible to give the chair an extra thrust with the arms at the crucial moment. Powered wheelchairs are not only very much heavier, they also usually have smaller wheels. Although one or two chairs like the Batricar can go up and down curbs quite easily, time may be taken to master the technique. In some areas, this may not be important. In country areas there frequently are no sidewalks and the wheelchair will use the road like any other vehicle. The obstacles will lie in the gradual gradients of the road, which a powered chair will manage very competently. In the town, curbs will present a problem in many cases. An alternative to trying to manage them is to try to use slopes instead: In an inner urban area these will occur at least where there are pedestrian crossings or garage or delivery entrances to factories or businesses. In suburban areas, convenient exits from garages will have to be found—unless the local authority is sufficiently enlightened to have introduced curb cuts, which are more generally for disabled users. Because of the limited range of the battery, it is unlikely that the wheelchair user will make a great variety of journeys within the mileage range, so the routes to be covered can be looked at carefully before buying, and a chair selected to suit the local environment. A child living on a farm and wishing to get across bumpy fields and up rough lanes will have quite different needs from the town child who wants to ride around the local shopping center or down a flat paved suburban pavement.

A further factor in choosing a chair may be the choice of steering available. If a child is severely disabled, it may be essential to choose a chair with power-assisted steering. Chair controls can be located on either arm of a chair for single-handed steering, or on a central column between the occupant's legs. The central control is usually convenient to use, but can make getting in and out of the chair rather awkward; and it can be a nuisance if a long skirt or cape is worn. Chairs like the Batricar overcome this problem by having the steering control far enough forward not to catch on any garments. An advantage of a steering column in the center for some wheelchair users is that it acts as a safety barrier, and makes it virtually impossible to fall forward out of the chair. On the other hand, a variety of safety straps can be purchased to provide safe anchorage in a powered chair with side controls.

If powered chairs are used all the time by a child who formerly used a manually operated chair, his arm muscles will not get the exercise to which they were formerly accustomed. This will mean that, without regular practice in a self-propelling chair, he will find it very difficult to change from a powered to a nonpowered chair in times of emergency when repairs or servicing is needed. Wheelchair users need to keep their shoulder and arm muscles as fit as possible, and it may be worth using a manual wheelchair for part of each day, however inconvenient it may be to have several wheelchairs in use around the house.

In conclusion, no powered chair should ever be purchased without a careful evaluation of its suitability. Most manufacturers are very willing to give demonstrations of their wheelchairs, and these can often be arranged at home. Wheelchairs can sometimes be purchased secondhand through journals or local magazines covering disability interests. Care should be taken when buying a secondhand chair, to make sure that it is in good condition and is, the appropriate size and model for the child; and chairs should never be purchased without a trial—mistakes can be expensive and very disappointing.

Using Powered Wheelchairs
Outside the Home

Many disabled people do not use a wheelchair extensively outside the home, and electric wheelchairs for indoor use are much lighter and more maneuverable than the heavier outdoor models. On the other hand, a wheelchair user in a country area or with many local social contacts will gain enormously from having a wheelchair like the Batricar, which will enable him to move about independently. If a child is approaching the age of legitimate driving, it may be worth balancing the purchase of an outdoor electric wheelchair against the cost of a modified car, since the latter offers less restricted transport.

If an independent electric wheelchair is purchased, it should be used with care on sidewalks and roads. As with bicycles, a single white lamp in front and single red lamp at the rear should be carried at night or in poor visibility. Some families experience opposition or even hostility from neighbors, who are alarmed at the sight of a tricycle or wheelchair moving along on the sidewalks. Road and sidewalk sense is essential, since the footrests or other parts of a wheelchair can deal a considerable blow to the unwary pedestrian. Some wheelchair users carry horns—although loud or blaring horns probably give other pedestrians a bigger fright than the actual chair. Nondisabled people, incidentally, can drive these powered wheelchairs and tricycles if they are taking them to or collecting them from a maintenance establishment. Since roads and pavements are congested in urban areas, this may be preferable to letting a relatively inexperienced teenager drive a powered chair through a busy town center. Road safety and experience are vital.

ATTACHMENTS AND ACCESSORIES

The suitability of most wheelchairs is made or marred by the range of attachments and accessories available to their users.

Brakes are important to stabilize the chair when out in the street, on a gradient, or for an attendant to operate when pushing a chair. Sometimes brake levers are difficult to reach without bending. Extension brake levers can then be fitted. Because permanent extension brake levers will make sideways transfer difficult on a wheelchair with removable arms, the levers may be detachable. Some wheelchairs which are designed as pushchairs have their brake levers on the pushing handles; others have foot brakes similar to those on carriage-type buggies. If elderly parents are going to push a heavy older child, they may like to take account of brake positions before finally selecting a chair. Some chairs have independent brakes (that is, on the left and right sides of the chair); others operate the braking system from a single lever. If the wheelchair user has to rely on one stronger arm, single lever brakes are the easiest to manage. They should, however, be checked periodically, as the use of a single lever tends to stretch the cable on one side, and the brakes may therefore start to work unevenly as the cable extends. If a wheelchair has pneumatic tires, attention should always be paid to the tire pressure, since the efficiency of the brakes may be slightly affected if the pressure becomes uneven or too low.

Wheels are usually a standard 20 in. (for the large rear wheels), but the size can be varied according to special needs. 22-in. and 24-in. wheels can be easier to reach and turn, as they offer better leverage, although they may form obstructions to sideways transfers out of or into the chair. Large wheels make tipping easier at curbs or other obstacles, but very large wheels are usually rather hard work to operate and to maneuver inside in a limited space. If a child has shortened or absent lower limbs, the usual large rear wheels may be dangerous, since they and the child's weight make the chair inclined to tip backward. In this case, the position of the wheels should be reversed, and the larger wheels put at the front. Not all wheelchairs can be modified in this way, and special advice should be sought. Sometimes the gravity problem can be overcome by fitting normal large rear propelling wheels further back than usual, so that the weight is more evenly distributed. It is usually easier to steer from the back, with the small front castors swiveling to change directions. Front-wheel–propelled chairs have two castors or sometimes a single castor at the back.

If a child has weak hands or shoulders, he may need additional support in propelling the wheels. A capstan handrim can be supplied on most wheelchairs. This is an inner handrim with eight spokes which can be pushed with the palm of the hand rather than with the whole hand and fingers, if necessary. One-arm propulsion wheels can also be prescribed and supplied on most wheelchairs. These require strong manual control in the good hand and take some skill to master. Physical therapists usually give basic instruction in propulsion and maneuvering.

Self-propelled chairs have two wheels and, usually, two castors. Castors are normally 5 in. in diameter and solid, but they can be varied on some chairs, with spokes for lightness or even with pneumatic tires for outdoor use. These modified castors are not as sturdy as the solid kind but may make a more comfortable ride. Large castors make steering more difficult but can make a chair more stable. Double castors are sometimes prescribed for large, heavy people, although the chair will require a bigger turning circle. Some front-propelled chairs have single rear castors, which make their turning circle very small in crowded areas like kitchens. This is convenient in an indoor chair, but less convenient outside where the chair would be less stable.

If a chair is to be used only as a pushed chair or is powered by an electric motor, big wheels are not necessary, and indeed will make the chair heavier and clumsier in movement. Most chairs have four wheels (which are easy to steer in a straight line), but some have two smaller wheels and two castors. The castors make a chair highly maneuverable in the house, but difficult to push straight along a pavement.

Backrests are important for comfort, particularly if there is some curvature (scoliosis) of the spine. Many folding chairs can be supplied with folding backrests, which fold down when the chair has to be loaded into a confined space such as a closet or the trunk of a car. Backrest extensions are available on some models, which give neck and head support. These can have side wings to give extra support to the head (particularly important with some cerebral palsied children who have little head control and need active support). If a chair is supplied with a fixed back, this can be adjusted at a suitable angle for individual use. Some chairs have adjustable backrests, and others have tilting mechanisms so that the position of the whole chair can be changed. These chairs are most useful for multiply or severely handicapped children.

Footrests are important for maintaining a good sitting position. When they are correctly adjusted (which is usually simply done with a spanner), the child's thighs should be horizontal on the seat, with the feet resting firmly in the rest. Many footrests are detachable and also hinged and retractable, which is useful for getting in and out of the chair. Children should be firmly discouraged from standing up with their feet in the footrests. Young children will sometimes try and reach something on a table or worktable by pushing down on the footrests and reaching up over the hard surface. Chairs will tip forward easily, particularly if there are large and heavy front wheels.

If footrests are easily removed (some can be detached by the individual in the wheelchair), the length of the chair is effectively shortened by about 8 to 9 in.–more if the footrests are extended to take braces. This can be useful when narrow places have to be negotiated. A number of special leg rests are supplied; these are detachable and meet the needs of children with limbs immobilized in plaster or in braces (when the leg usually has to be held straight). They can also be used to elevate the legs into a semireclining position, if this is required for any reason. A variety of extra fittings, such as toe loops, check straps, and heel restraining loops, are available to keep the feet in place. Toes dragging on the ground, or catching on castors, are uncomfortable and potentially dangerous.

Some chairs have removable *armrests*; these are essential if the wheelchair user wishes to make sideway transfers in the bathroom or bedroom, and are often necessary for sitting comfortably at a desk or table. Nonfolding chairs with rigid arms can sometimes be supplied with domestic armrests. These are cut out so that the seat of the chair can project under a work surface. Everest and Jennings' chairs (which have some of the widest ranges of accessories and personal modifications) have desk arms with cutouts at the rear for *ball-bearing arm supports.* Arm supports are necessary when arm control is weak or the muscles go into spasms. The supports balance the forearms, allowing them to move freely and horizontally, with a downward movement to drop the hand to reach down to a working surface to write or pick up food. They should be carefully adjusted, since the ball-bearing swivels with minimum movement and careful adjustment can give fine control of hand movement. If the supports are not properly adjusted, the arms will move around uselessly.

Many children like to have a tray attachment to their chair. This can be fitted to most children's models and is useful for eating, working, or playing. Tray attachments can vary between straightforward trays that fit close to the body and molded, plastic-lipped trays that hold toys and utensils and prevent them from falling onto the floor.

Cushions are very important to people in wheelchairs and can be supplied through appliance centers. They should be ordered by the doctor making the recommendation for the wheelchair. Wheelchair cushions vary in thickness (usually from 1 to 4 in.) and should be selected to match the height of the seat and armrests of the individual chair. Deep, soft cushions may look comfortable, but they often further incapacitate a severely handicapped person who sinks into them and cannot easily move. If a child is paraplegic or is in any way at risk from pressure sores (particularly when immobilized after surgery or fractures), ripple cushions may be best. Inflatable air cushions, gel cushions, or "bean bags" stuffed with polystyrene granules are also useful. Some children find medical sheepskins comfortable, which certainly help the problem of perspiration and discomfort which comes from sitting on plastic or leatherette surfaces for long periods of time. If a child needs to make sliding transfers from a chair, cushions should be chosen which permit an easy transition. A foam cushion covered with leatherette on a plywood base may be both comfortable and convenient for sliding.

Special *paraplegic cushions* are also available, which can incorporate a urinal. Chair seats can also be fitted with commode facilities. In one model, the plywood base with an aperture has a removable covered cushion, so that the wheelchair can be wheeled directly over the toilet when the sitting cushion has been removed; while another model incorporates latex cushions with a permanently exposed aperture. These models are not normally appropriate for children, though they can be used for adolescents if required. Generally sanichairs or commode chairs are more appropriate than commode facilities incorporated into a chair. The paraplegic cushion, on the other hand, which has a U-shape cut out of the front for the insertion of a urinal, may be useful for older children who wish to be independent and who can manage the independent use of a urinal. It can also be very useful when a heavy child is temporarily incapacitated by a cast or surgery, and access to the toilet is difficult.

When children are severely physically handicapped, with major abnormalities of the spine or posture, sitting comfortably may be very difficult without further aggravating their handicap. Molded seat shells by Desemo, Inc., have recently been developed. The child is seated in the best postural position in a large rubber bag containing polystyrene beads and epoxy resin. When he is moved away, this is used as a mold to vacuum-form a thermoplastic seat shell with a liner that fits the child's body. The shell is fitted onto a base board and can then be fitted into a wheelchair or other chair. A molded toilet seat can be made in the same way.

Whatever type of chair is used, many children will require safety straps to ensure that they do not fall about in or out of their chairs. A wide range of seat belts are available that can be adjusted to wheelchair or car use. Children with cerebral palsy or multiple handicaps may have strong muscle spasms, which make postural control difficult. Groin and shoulder straps are available for most models, and care should be taken that they are adjusted well, so that the child is supported in the best position and not imprisoned in a thoroughly uncomfortable one.

Weatherproof aprons are available for most outdoor models, if required. Alternatively, protective clothing can be worn. Some outdoor chairs like the Batricar can be supplied with miniature "cabins" to protect the occupant from rain or wind. These larger chairs are expensive but give considerable freedom to older children and young people outside the home.

Maintenance of Wheelchairs

Wheelchairs, like bicycles and motorcars, benefit from regular maintenance and routine care. A wheelchair which is used entirely inside the house and is seldom folded or moved will obviously suffer much less wear and tear than a wheelchair which is used inside and out, and which is frequently folded up and moved around in a car trunk.

All wheelchairs should be carefully and routinely checked over. Brakes are most important. If these are inadequate (and the chair and its occupant can be very heavy), the chair may run away if left outside a store or on a sloping sidewalk. Equally, if brakes are inadequate and the disabled person starts to get up and move off the chair, the chair may tilt and move forward. It is extremely difficult for a disabled person to recover his balance, and a tipping wheelchair is a heavy object to have fall on top of you on the floor. It is always wise make sure. The front castors need to be fully mobile, but often become tangled up with pieces of cotton or woolen thread from the carpet. If they are not completely free, the wheelchair is difficult to push and will not steer properly.

Tire pressure is important on a wheelchair with pneumatic tires. Very hard or very soft tires make the wheelchair more difficult to operate. If tire pressure is constantly going down, the valves may need attention. Local garages and bicycle shops usually do this kind of minor servicing with reasonable speed and at a moderate cost. Remember that tire pressures will seem much higher when the chair is empty. A heavy adolescent with braces will place a great amount of weight on the chair, and pressure needs to take account of this additional weight. Tire pressure gauges can be purchased quite cheaply and are a simple way of checking.

Chrome and other metal work should be kept clean and dry if exposed to rain or bad weather. Tires can become very muddy and accumulate bits of grass, twigs, and garden debris if a chair is used inside and out. Wheelchair tires, like stroller tires, can be kept partially clean by installing a large, nonslip, rough-textured mat in the porch or entrance. Because wheelchairs tend to get caught in loose material or mats, it is safest if this is recessed into the floor to give an even level, or if it is secured in some way. If the same chair is used outside and inside, it is sensible to have a tough washable surface in the hall so that carpets are not spoiled and tempers are not worsened with constant trails of dirt!

Handrims are important on self-propelled wheelchairs. These can become loose and wobbly. They should be regularly checked and tightened. Suitable tools can be purchased from do-it-yourself shops, and in some cases are supplied by the manufacturers of the chair.

If the wheelchair has an instruction book, follow its maintenance hints carefully. Instruction books give details about the timing and extent of oiling of ballbearing and other joints. Follow the instructions; too much oil will probably spread to the upholstery, fingers, and other furnishings and will not achieve any purpose. The upholstery of the wheelchair should be treated according to the manufacturer's instructions. Usually sponging and drying will be all that is necessary. Chair upholstery is often damaged by overzealous helpers who try to fold the chair incorrrectly. Make sure that the chair is not folded up with the seat cushion still inside. Wheelchairs should never be lifted by their arm rests (which will usually come away), and any movable parts such as footrests or headrests should be neatly stacked when the chair is stored, and not allowed to be knocked over or damaged. Storage can be a problem if several wheelchairs have to be kept in a small apartment or house, and damage can sometimes occur because a chair is forced into a closet, or is stacked with other heavy objects. This is particularly likely to happen to a second chair that is used only occasionally. If the chair has special sheepskin or ripple cushions, these should be cleaned and cared for according to the supplier's instructions. Many sheepskins are washable in pure detergent and warm water. They should never be dried in front of electric heaters or on radiators, or they will harden and crack.

Damage sometimes occurs because the chair is mishandled when folded and lifted in and out of the car trunk. The easiest way to lift a chair into a car trunk is to place the folded chair close to and parellel with the trunk of the car. The chair should be picked up by gripping convenient struts of the chair—never wheels, armrests, or other movable parts. The chair is then lifted vertically and balanced on the edge of the trunk (if this is high and has a sharp "lip," a car rug can be placed over it to avoid snags and tears). The chair is then tipped until nearly horizontal, with the wheels taking the weight on the edge of the trunk, and when nearly horizontal slid in. Even the lightest of chairs can be heavy, particularly if the car trunk is small. If a helper is available, there is less risk of damage or jolting. Removable parts should be placed inside *after* the chair, not under it. Swivel arm rests and some other extra parts are quite delicate and can be badly bent if a chair is pushed in on top of them.

The regular wheelchair users—the family—will quickly develop strategies to move wheelchairs around, but enthusiastic helpers are inclined to do damage if not closely observed the first time. Electric folding chairs, in particular, need careful attention because of the necessity to manage the battery. Manufacturer's instructions should be very carefully followed, and it may be advisable to return the chair to the manufacturer for periodic servicing. Arrangements for any special servicing should be discussed before purchasing, as facilities may vary throughout the country.

REPAIRS AND MAINTENANCE

Wheelchairs are precision instruments—and like all mechanical objects they will sometimes break down. A British survey of wheelchairs and their users found that 13 percent (12,500 wheelchairs) of all the wheelchairs in the survey were in need of some kind of repair at the time of interview. While this may indicate that wheelchair service is not entirely satisfactory in maintaining chairs in good condition, it may also reflect on the reluctance of families to let a wheelchair go for repair until it is in need of drastic treatment.

It is very important to find out *in advance* how to bridge the gap with a temporary chair, and to obtain precise information on how repairs will be dealt with when the need occurs. Additionally it should be remembered that some of the most sophisticated powered chairs require very expert attention, and the waiting may therefore be longest for those who have the greatest need and the most limited access to other mobility aids. A wheelchair loaned as a stopgap may not be as satisfactory as the usual chair, but it is essential to have an emergency procedure for ensuring that a child (particularly a large child who is too heavy to carry) is not immobilized or even bed-bound while a wheelchair is being repaired.

If minor repairs (like punctures or small adjustments) are required, the chair can be taken to a local garage or cycle shop. This is usually a much quicker procedure. Some families do quite elaborate repairs to their own chairs at home. If they have experience and the right tools, this may be useful, economical, and bypass a good deal of delay and inconvenience. However, care should be taken with home repairs. Also, it is of course potentially dangerous to tamper with brakes or the basic structure of the chair. Brakes and tires are the parts most likely to become faulty, together with batteries on electric chairs. Tires can often be dealt with at home, but brakes should be dealt with only carefully and with expert advice.

INSTRUCTIONS ON USING A CHAIR

Wheelchairs, like cars, have their own individual characteristics and temperaments. It is very important that a chair's use should be *demonstrated* and that parents and child should be quite clear about folding, movement, fitting, and removal of any armrests, headrests, and so forth. It should be standard procedure to receive an instruction booklet with the chair. However, a British survey found that over three quarters of the wheelchair users questioned (79 percent) claimed that no instruction booklets had ever been received. Memories can be faulty, but 72 percent of wheelchair users who had acquired a new chair in the previous twelve months could also not recall receiving any instruction booklet.

An instruction booklet should contain basic information on general care and maintenance of the chair, details of its operation and folding procedure, mechanical details, and how to get repairs. Parents may feel, if they have had a demonstration of a chair, that they do not need any superfluous bits of paper. But booklets are always useful for reference and, even if not looked at again for several years, can give practical advice on any minor mechanical failures or on general care. It is best that the booklet be *requested* as soon as the chair is ordered. Parents should remember to *ask* and to ensure that they also know what arrangements are to be made for any minor repairs. Instruction books are particularly important with powered wheelchairs and with a very severely handicapped child whose chair is usually pushed by an attendant rather than self-propelled. Parents become very adept at manipulating a heavy wheelchair up and down curbs, and at folding and fitting any attachment. Other relatives or friends may not appreciate the danger of not using a tipping lever on curbs or may fix leg and arm attachments incorrectly. It is sensible to show them written information first to avoid scares or (much worse) accidents.

If a child is attending a wheelchair clinic, he will certainly have an opportunity to test the chair and have its general mechanical operation demonstrated before taking it home. Demonstrations are the most effective form of instruction—most of us do not read printed instructions carefully enough! If a child is attending a wheelchair clinic, it may be useful if both his parents attend with him, so that they also can ask questions about the wheelchair's operation and care. If a chair is being selected for use with an attendant, it is particularly important that the attendant not only comment on the choice of a chair (convenience of height of handles, weight, and so forth), but also see the chair properly used in action. The center is not intended to operate as an instruction center for the person receiving the chair (although some centers do offer a good deal of useful advice). It is therefore important to *request* advice from the physical therapist or occupational therapist in the local hospital (preferably through the wheelchair clinic if this is available).

If a child attends a special school, he will normally receive instruction in manipulating a chair and will be encouraged to use the chair as a genuine mobility aid for a variety of activities. Ironically, some of the potentially most capable wheelchair users may never receive this instruction (because they are moving in more integrated settings), and may have great difficulties in mastering curbs and some of the finer maneuvers which are very difficult in a wheelchair. If this is a problem, membership in a local physically handicapped sporting or other club may be useful to acquire optimum skills. Wheelchair sports or wheelchair dancing (which was designed as an educational aid to greater flexibility in wheelchair use) will also encourage experiment for the wheelchair child. However knowledge and practical experience of the use of a wheelchair are acquired, one should ask for all necessary information immediately to ensure that maximum independence is achieved. Learning to use a wheelchair can be very difficult in the beginning and particularly tiring for the more severely or newly handicapped. It is essential that children are not discouraged and that parents do not get into the habit of pushing the chair unnecessarily, thus (indirectly) discouraging its use because the child's first attempts are so slow and clumsy around the house.

HINTS FOR WHEELCHAIR USERS
AND HELPERS

There are many different types of wheelchairs, and they all have their own "personalities" according to the model, accessories, and general design. Both users and helpers should familiarize themselves with instructions about brakes, folding, maneuvering, and so forth. These instructions should accompany the chair and if not supplied should be requested direct from the manufacturer or from the appliance center.

It is very important to check that the brakes are on, whether getting into a chair independently or with helpers. Chairs are more stable if backed against a wall or another piece of furniture. If the armrests are removable, it is often convenient to remove them on one or both sides when transferring a disabled child to a chair. It is never wise to try to move a chair with removable armrests by its arms, or to pick it up by the arms. If the armrests come away, the chair may be damaged and (if the child is sitting in it) may tip over and fall. When the child is getting out of the chair, it is absolutely essential not to allow him to start to get up or stand on the footrests. Even if the chair is front-wheel propelled, it will tend to tip forward. Disabled children usually have difficulty in reacting quickly to an emergency situation and may fall heavily. Many footrests swivel around or are detachable, and may have to be moved before the occupant gets up.

Even if a wheelchair is self-propelled, a child may need help with a curb, garden step, or other obstacle. When a wheelchair is pushed *down* over an obstacle, the tipping lever on the chair is operated by the attendant so that the chair is tipped backwards. As the large rear wheels go down, some of the chair's weight is taken by the attendant. Care should be taken to hold both handles and distribute the weight equally. If one large wheel goes down before the other, the chair can be unstable and may tip. Some people find it easier to back a chair down a curb. Once the back wheels are down, the front wheels can be lowered and the chair can go forward.

Getting a wheelchair *up* and over an obstacle is more difficult. The chair is tipped by the tipping lever onto its rear wheels. The front wheels then ride up on the curb. If a chair is very heavy or the obstacle very high, it may be necessary to have a helper. Helpers should not pull on the arm or footrests (which may be damaged or come away) but should lift from the front wheels. Many wheelchair users are able to give a thrust on the rear wheels to help, and the chair will mount easily. It is necessary not to run the chair hard up against the curb, since the castors will then serve as an obstacle and force will simply tip the chair. Wheelchairs can be lifted up flights of steps, but two helpers are needed for this. They should understand what they are doing as the chair will have to be tipped back onto its large rear wheels and brought up in this position. It is particularly important not to put weight on removable parts of the chair. If in doubt, it is better to take the chair and child up separately. The principles used are basically those needed to pull a buggy up steps: Most mothers of young children will not find this difficult, but others may! Going downstairs is potentially much more dangerous, and a child may need to be strapped in. Many disabled children find it painful to be "bumped" up or down stairs, and it may be better to carry them separately.

Many good helpers forget to listen to the disabled person himself. He usually knows how the chair works—but even grandmothers and grandfathers can be overconfident. Clothes, rugs, and so forth can all catch in wheels if not properly positioned. Legs, particularly in paraplegic children, need to be watched, as the child may have no sensation in his lower limbs and may not notice rubbing. Brothers and sisters sometimes forget that they are not taking part in a rodeo. Of course, disabled children enjoy games like anybody else—but they can be frightened if chairs are bumped, jerked, or stopped and started too rapidly. A small child in a buggy is seated facing his mother and can anticipate changes of direction or speed. A child in a wheelchair is facing straight ahead. Speed can be terrifying if the chair is apparently making headlong progress over a busy road without stopping, or if the child's feet, arms, or (worst for the victim) hard parts of the chair are banged into unwary pedestrians. Disabled people will not endear themselves to their neighbors if their chair catches unwary shins or ankles—and attendants do sometimes misjudge distances.

LIFTING IN AND OUT
OF THE WHEELCHAIR

Small disabled people or children do not usually present great problems when lifting is required. Larger or heavier handicapped people may cause great difficulty, particularly if the helpers concerned are inexperienced and uncertain what to do. When the disabled person can take some weight on his feet, the easiest method of transfer from the wheelchair is for the helper to arch his back (to avoid strain), place his feet so that the child's feet are controlled and will not fly out or slip, and put his arms around the helper's back and neck, he can be lifted into an upright position. He can then be "walked" to the seat or chair. When two helpers are available, and when the child is severely handicapped or very heavy a variety of shoulder lifts can be used. The helpers place their arms under the child's armpits from front to back. Their outside arms are used to steady his back and push his hips straight. The helpers should grasp hands to equalize their hold. Variations on this hold include supporting the child under the knees, or sharing the weight between one helper supporting the child under the arms and the other around the waist or under the legs. Care should be taken in lifting very severely handicapped children, since bones or joints can easily be damaged by clumsy or inappropriate handling. If possible it is preferable to ask a physical therapist to demonstrate, and (ideally) to include any relatives involved in the care of the child in the demonstration. District nurses, who frequently have to move heavy elderly people single-handed, are also useful sources of advice.

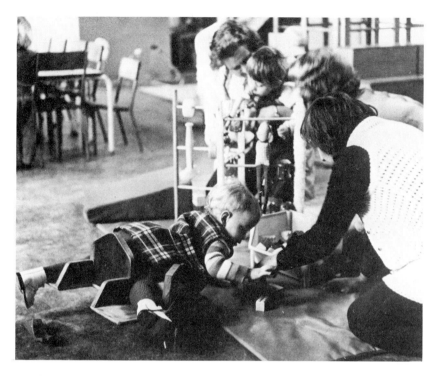

Learning to play out of the wheelchair at the Opportunity Class, Stevenage. *Copyright G. D. Clark and National Children's Bureau.*

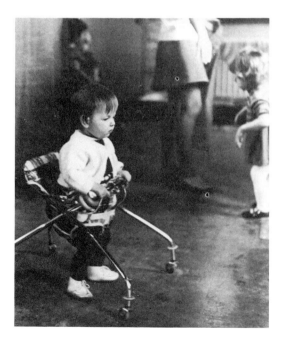

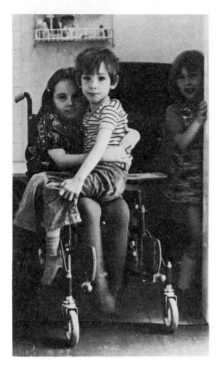

Handicap is a family affair. With a little help, the handicapped child in a wheelchair can join in family life and even help look after the able-bodied brothers and sisters. *Copyright G. D. Clark and National Children's Bureau.*

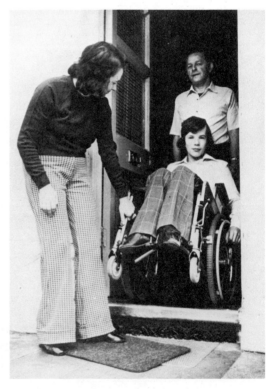

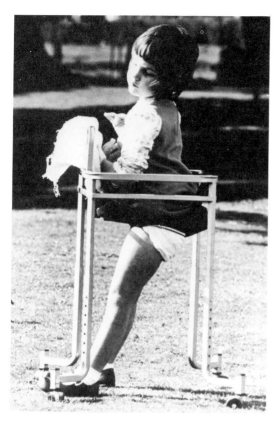

Walker frames can help young children to enjoy the garden and outdoor play. *Copyright G. D. Clark and National Children's Bureau.*

Outdoor mobility in the Batricar. *Copyright Associated Newspapers Group Limited.*

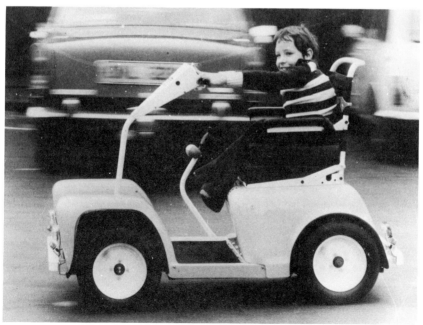

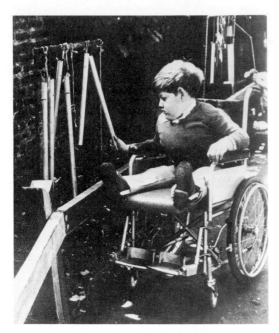

Handicapped Adventure Playgrounds in the U. K. provide supervised play, ensuring that challenge is combined with safety and responsible risk taking. Handicapped children can enjoy the normal outside activities of able-bodied children. Even bonfires and baked potatoes are possible! *Copyright Camilla Jessel.*

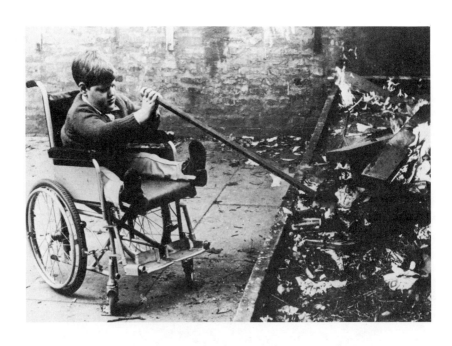

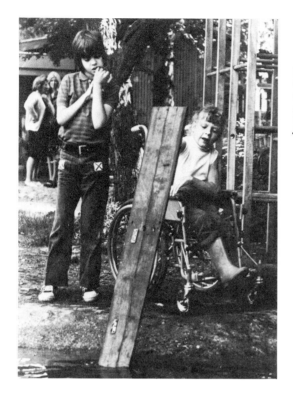

Handicapped children
enjoy shared activities
and games–particularly
getting wet and muddy!
*Copyright Camilla
Jessel.*

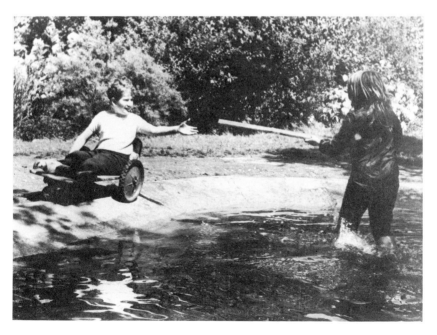

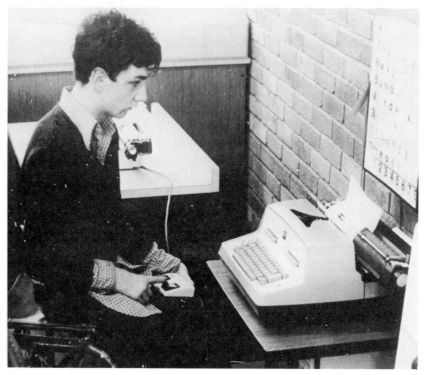

Specialized equipment such as a possum typewriter can help to overcome communication problems. Photographed at Banstead Place, Banstead, Surrey, U. K. *Copyright Queen Elizabeth Foundation for the Disabled.*

Teenage students at Banstead Place have the opportunity to learn how to look after themselves for two weeks or more in a self-contained bedsitting room. Handicapped adolescents need considerable help and encouragement to become fully independent. *Copyright Queen Elizabeth Foundation for the Disabled.*

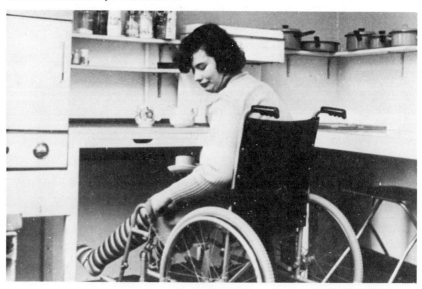

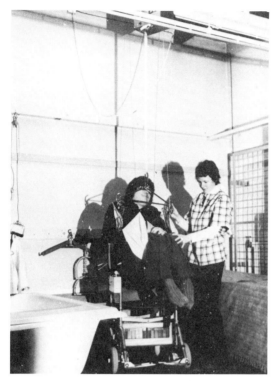

Independent living often means using hoists and other mechanical aids. At Barnstead Place an occuaptional therapist instructs a young student in the use of a hoist for transfer from wheelchair to bath. Copyright *Queen Elizabeth Foundation for the Disabled.*

A student working in her study bedroom at Ullenwood Manor College of Further Education. Many handicapped students gain from a period in a special college or assessment center before going on to higher education or to open employment. *Copyright National Star Centre for Disabled Youth, Ullenwood, Gloucestershire, U. K.*

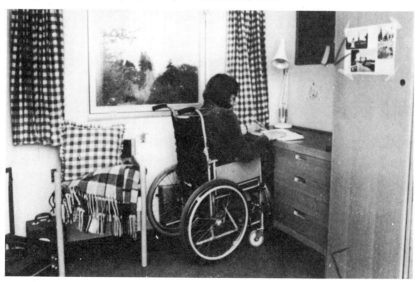

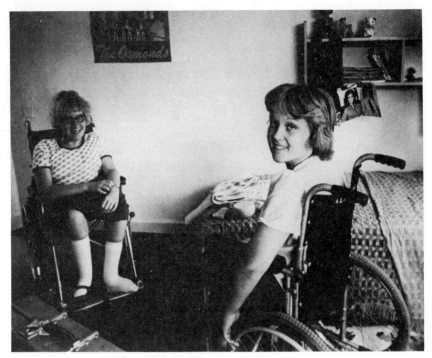

Going away from home can open new horizons and develop new friendships. Two students at the National Star Centre meet for a chat in one of the study bedrooms at Ullenwood Manor. *Copyright National Star Centre for Disabled Youth.*

Many people in wheelchairs enjoy sports. Students at Ullenwood Manor practice archery for a forthcoming sports event. *Copyright National Star Centre for Disabled Youth.*

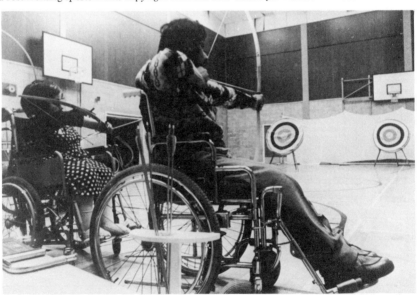

7

The Cost
of Disability

DAY-TO-DAY LIVING:
MANAGING AT HOME

Living with a handicap can be expensive. Studies of families with a
handicap member have found that the actual *additional* cost is difficult to estimate. We live in a consumer-oriented society, in which,
in city areas in particular, it is generally accepted that the wife will
return to work and supplement the family income as her children get
older and more independent. This is also reflected, in part, by the
increasing number of one-parent families, which include many
families where there is a handicapped child. And this loss of income
is one of the first sacrifices that families with a handicapped child
often have to make. It is perhaps assumed too easily that parents can
and will cope. And indeed, most parents do wish to care for their
handicapped child at home. But they have to face a great deal,

143

including the loss of the wife's income (if she had otherwise expected to work), and all the additional travel, heating, clothing, and other costs of caring for a handicapped child.

Expense with a handicapped child is an ongoing affair. A study of wheelchair users (*The Extra Cost of Disabled Living*, Mavis Hyam Action Research for the Crippled Child, U. K., 1977), found that living in a wheelchair brought about a 20 to 25 percent increase in total household expenses. The fifty-six wheelchair users in the study (who were of working age, but whose problems were common to younger age groups) all had expenses related to heating, clothing, laundry, and supplies from the druggist. The report particularly emphasized the loss of family income when one member of that family could not work because special care was needed by the disabled person.

SUPPLEMENTARY SECURITY INCOME

Supplementary Security Income (SSI) is a federal income maintenance program for disabled persons. It is administered by the Social Security Administration in each state. This program provides monthly payments to those who have little or no income.

Eligible individuals must be children with a serious visual impairment or other disability, or adults who are over 65 years of age or are blind or disabled and have a limited income and resources.

A child who has a physical or mental impairment may qualify for these benefits. To qualify, the diagnosis must be of a handicap that is comparable in severity to one which would incapacitate an adult for at least 12 months or result in death.

Since these benefits are based on need as well as disability, the parents' income and resources are used to figure eligibility. The maximum benefit at present, subject to changes in pending federal legislation and changes in the cost of living index, is $304.30 per month.

A further benefit for SSI recipients is Medicaid. Those individuals designated as eligible for SSI benefits are also eligible to receive Medicaid benefits.

Application for SSI should be made to your local Social Security office. The determination of eligibility is based on an individual basis. Your local office will assign a representative to your case and help you secure the benefits if you are entitled to them.

FEDERAL INCOME TAX

In order to reduce the tax burden on people with disabilities and their families, a number of rules have been included to assist in filing income tax deductions.

A major area of concern to parents of physically handicapped individuals is medical care. Medical care—including payments for diagnosis, prevention and treatment, and fees to health care practitioners—can be deducted. Also included in medical deductions are operations, prescription drugs, and over-the-counter drugs prescribed or recommended by a physician. Special services can also be included. These are hospital and laboratory fees, ambulance services, and nursing assistance at home. If special aids are required for your disabled child the cost is also deductible. This includes mechanical devices, special furniture, special telephone equipment, wheelchairs, and so on. All transportation costs that are related to medical care are also deductible. The standard mileage rate is nine cents per mile.

The parent of a disabled child may also claim a dependent exemption of $1,000. Even if the dependent lives in a medical facility or nursing home, they may be claimed if five basic criteria are met:

1. The parent, i.e., tax payer, must pay more than half the dependent's support.
2. The dependent must not have a gross income of $1,000 or more unless he/she is a child under 19 years of age.
3. The dependent must be a member of the household or a relative.
4. The dependent must be a United States citizen, resident, or national.
5. The dependent cannot file a joint tax return on his own.

Child care credit is also available to parents of handicapped or disabled dependents. Specific income-related ceilings for credit are used, so questions should be addressed to your local Internal Revenue Service office.

In order to be prepared to file a tax return to utilize these deductions it is essential for individuals to keep careful records. All expenses related to your child's disability should be recorded, including date of payment, name and address of person providing the service, brief description of the service, amount paid, and if possible, a receipt. Records should be kept for a minimum of three years.

8

The Physical Environment

ADAPTING LIVING AREAS

Obviously parents (and their handicapped children) will wish to maintain their homes as "homes" and not as hospitals. But certain common-sense considerations need to be paid to reorganizing the house for a family member with a mobility problem. Wheelchairs take room, especially when turning, and living areas need space for access. Nonslip and hard-wearing floor coverings are best. Cord or cork tiles wear well and look attractive. Some of the textured carpets are difficult to push a chair over, but the degree of mobility of the occupant is relevant. Loose rugs may look pretty but should be avoided. They are easily entangled in wheelchair wheels, make pushing more difficult, and (most importantly) are liable to be rolled up by the wheelchair so that other members of the family may fall and hurt themselves. An important safety factor is the positioning of electric lights and plugs. Switches may need to be repositioned at a lower level for a wheelchair child. Special switches can be obtained which respond to a very light touch; table lamps should be carefully positioned to avoid accidents; and switches for stereo equipment, heat, and so forth are safest at waist height.

Anybody using a wheelchair is likely to notice the cold more than an active able-bodied person. Some form of central heating is the ideal and safe way of providing background heating, but a handicapped person may need extra heat in certain areas of the house. Kerosene heaters are very dangerous for anybody with impaired mobility. Although the new models are self-extinguishing, they are still a hazard because of the risk of spilling the oil. If they must be used, they should be fastened to the wall and protected by a suitable guard. Because of the lack of sensation in their legs, many handicapped people will be very much at risk of burns or scorches. A large fireguard will keep limbs at a safe distance from the source of heat. Gas fires are useful and economical methods of heating a room, but controls should be looked at carefully. If electric heaters are used, they should be fastened to the wall, or in panels fixed into the plaster. Small electric heaters are a potential hazard of their light weight and ease of tipping.

GETTING INTO THE HOUSE

Doorways are constant sources of difficulty for wheelchair users. To allow for a wheelchair, the recommended minimum opening required is 79 cm (31 in.). This opening leaves little room for maneuvering, and a door of 84 cm a (33 in.) is preferable. A wheelchair user will find it helpful to have a handle or bar at a suitable height to pull and push the door open and shut, although the easiest door to operate is a sliding door with top and bottom runners. If this is not possible, access to a difficult or angled door can sometimes be made easier by rehanging the door to open in the opposite direction. Raised thresholds are a problem to wheelchairs negotiating a narrow opening and should be leveled if possible.

When a child is old enough to be left alone in the house, it is useful to think of safety precautions for the front door. Glass peepholes are widely available—or it may be possible to fit a mirror in a room that shows the child who is calling without allowing the child to be seen. If the child finds it difficult to get to the front door quickly, an intercom system might be considered. The caller rings the bell and the occupant picks up an internal telephone receiver and asks who it is. If the answer is acceptable, the door is opened by remote control through a push button.

For the severely disabled, electrically operated doors are available. These can be operated by a photocell light beam or by contact. The contact can be triggered off by a variety of factors, including pull-strings or buttons. The installation of equipment like this is extremely expensive, and is unlikely to be generally available.

RAMPS

Ramps are necessary for a wheelchair to transfer between levels. All ramps must have a gradual slope in order to enable the wheelchair to be propelled or pushed safely without risk of accident. If the area to be negotiated is very steep and short, a series of shallow steps may be more negotiable. The wheelchair is taken up each step as up a curb. Once the wheelchair reaches the top of the gradient, a flat space is needed in front of the door or gate. This can often be accommodated by an existing porch. Ramps that are very narrow can be dangerous: Many wheelchairs are heavy, and there is the risk that one wheel may come off the ramp and tip the chair over. All ramps should have adequate handrails, and these should extend at least 1 ft (305 mm) at each end of the ramp. Handrails, if fixed to a wall, should give good clearance for a hand grasping them (in practice usually about 1¾ in. (44 mm). They should be secure and easy to grip, with brackets fixed to the underside of the rail. The wheelchair attendant also needs a handrail of about 39 in. in height (991 mm). Wheelchair users need a lower height of about 30 in. (762 mm). A compromise height can be used, but if a chair is often propelled by a tall attendant, it may be better to have double rails.

If access to a yard with a number of levels is required, or if there are delays in having ramps installed, outside ramps can be made quite simply at home. There are many movable ramps on the market. The "Expamet" ramp is made of metal and can be bolted onto an existing step. It can be unbolted and moved as required. Lightweight portable ramps are available to be carried on a wheelchair. The Amigo curb ramp with hinged center can be attached to the back of the seat for convenience. These can be used on curbs or steps. As they are useless unless all the wheels and castors are in line and the ramp must be picked up and put down as necessary, they require full use of arm, shoulder, and body muscles. The lightweight portable wheelchair ramps manufactured by Simcross fold and can mount a step up to 8 in. (203 mm) high. They are strong enough to take an electric wheelchair, and extra long ramps are also available. Rootes manufactures portable ramps that are similar in design. The "Porta-ramp" is very lightweight, made of fiberglass, and can mount two steps. Tyrpod makes safety ramps that are very useful in houses. These ramps consist of a number of solid rubber-ridged sections that lock together to form a ramp. They can also be carried for use on outside steps or curbs. The type of wheelchair, weight and ability of the child, and the cost of the sections make advance planning before purchase advisable.

ELECTRIC LIFTS

Stairclimbers

As a child gets bigger, lifting him up and down stairs can become a major problem. The answer can be the installation of a stair-climber or a lift. Stairclimbers are easy to install and require little in the way of building alterations. They are electrically operated and have cut-off devices for any electrical or other failure. The majority of stair-climbers ride up the side of the stairs, leaving space for normal use.

Stairlifts

Since a wheelchair user will need two wheelchairs if he is obliged to leave his chair on the ground floor, the more disabled will find stair-lifts for wheelchair and occupant more useful than a climber. These stairlifts operate on a platform principle, with the lift mounting on two channels. The lift motor can normally be placed under the stairs. A wheelchair stairlift will require more structural alterations than a climber, since a pit or ramp must be created in order for the lift to reach ground level. The type of stairlift selected also depends upon the type of staircase, since special tracks are needed to accommodate bends or curves in the stairs.

Traditional Lifts

Traditional *lifts* require more structural adaptations and greater expense and planning in their installation. The simplest lift, such as the home lift manufactured by Wessex, is a conventional enclosed lift car that runs on two guide rails bolted to the wall. The lift goes through a trap opening in the ceiling. Some lifts can be balanced and hand-driven. The wheelchair and occupant travel on an open platform, with the mechanism operated by either the wheelchair passenger or a second person.

A number of firms manufacture hydraulic lifts which are platform lifts covering short rises. These are useful for covering a flight of steep steps between the road and the front door, or in split-level houses, where there is insufficient space for ramps. They are usually electrically operated, working on a scissor-type mechanism which is housed under the platform. Hydraulic lifts usually have a range of about 1.8 m (6 ft).

The selection of a particular lift depends upon a number of variables. An occupational therapist can give helpful advice. However, the potential hazard of a stairlift to other occupants of the house, or the inconvenience of the lift mechanism and trap in a living room, may also enter into consideration. Needless to say, lifts should be treated with the greatest respect and attention to safety. Not only are regular checks necessary for the sake of the handicapped person, but also for the safety of other members of the family. Small children play on stairs and find electrical gadgets irresistible. Lifts are not toys, and the kind of safety barriers and gates provided for trapdoors in a normal home will not be as childproof as those used in hotels and offices.

SPECIAL FURNITURE

Many children will use their wheelchairs for normal sitting activities within the family home. Their needs will, therefore, not be specifically considered in relation to the general furnishings in the living area, though it would be as well to make sure that these furnishings are secure, firm, and not easily damaged by knocks and bumps. If however the child wishes to get out of his wheelchair and use a more normal chair, there are a range of special designs to choose from. Most modern armchairs are low, with sloping backs, and are uncomfortable for severely handicapped people. They are also too low for easy transfer to and from the wheelchair or walking aid.

There are a number of chairs that have spring-lifted seats, and more elaborate chairs have a mechanical or electric lifting mechanism, but both require that the chair's occupant be able to put enough weight on his feet to lean forward. They can also be dangerous if the lift is too sudden for the severity of the occupant's disability. An exception is the "riser" chair, which is operated by electricity and which lifts the chair arms with the seat, so that the sitter is slowly raised to his feet. This type of chair is expensive, and is unlikely to be necessary or supplied for a child. It can, however, be very useful for some disabled adolescents.

If the child has stiff hips, he may wish his chair to be angled for a distribution of weight forward rather than backward. This can often be achieved by shortening the front legs, so that the sitting position is comfortable and easy to alter. Care should be taken in shortening legs or altering the weight distribution of standard chairs, since the alteration in stress may make them dangerous in time. Handicapped people are in any case frequently heavy users of furniture, because they need to lean and push to a much greater extent than able-bodied people.

Tables should, in particular, be stable and the correct height to avoid accidents. There are a number of special tables for handicapped children who can only stand in braces. These can also be made at home by cutting out one or more semicircular pieces from a table of suitable height. Adapted tables can be purchased from a number of suppliers. J. A. Preston manufactures a play table which enables four children to play together. The table has four cutouts. Large tables like this may seem expensive, but they have the great advantage of offering opportunities for group play. As the legs are adjustable, the table can grow with the child. This is an important factor in balancing the cost of a homemade adaptation of an old coffee or kitchen table (which will be grown out of fairly quickly) against the cost of an adaptable model. Preston also makes a useful individual play or school table which is covered with scratch-resistant plastic and has a rim around. The table can be used by the child in a wheelchair and had adjustable legs. It should be remembered that children seated in a wheelchair will need a different height of table when they are standing in braces.

If economy is essential, or if an outdoor play table is required, a simple and cheap standing table can be made from an old table (perhaps purchased in a garage sale). Provided the table is stable and its legs are strong, a circular hole of about 12 in. can be cut in the center. The legs are then cut so that the table is approximately the chest-height of the child when standing. If the edges of the hole are then padded with foam, with plastic, the child can be lifted into the hole and can stand supported. The useful life of this table is, of course, limited for a young growing child, since it will give proportionately less support as he grows; it is also hard work lifting a large child weighted with braces over the table and into the hole. The advantage is that a play table is manufactured very simply and cheaply; many children like an old table in the garden (where they can use clay, papier-maché, poster paints, and so forth, with impunity). It is usually sensible to put a wooden trim around the table to prevent toys falling off. If the table is left outside or used for messy games, it may be necessary to bore small holes in the beading so that water can drain off when the table is cleaned. A wooden table can be painted with blackboard paint, so that it can be directly chalked or painted on. If a child has coordination problems, the use of such a table can avoid a good deal of mess and recrimination. Again, the size of the average kitchen table will leave plenty of space for communal games if necessary: One small boy successfully utilized such a table for an electric railway layout. He stood in the center organizing his track and operating the transformer, while his friends stood around the outside. Although lifting him in presented some problems, he was able to play without risk of falling and breaking his models, and he was easily able to play with neighborhood friends.

If a child is to enjoy a variety of games and play experiences, it may be important to look at the very wide range of material available and experiment with chairs, cushions, and foam pads. The "Suzy" chair (see Appendix B for manufacturer) is an inflatable chair resembling a shell. When inflated, it can be used in the bath, on the beach, or in the house. It needs support, and can be jammed between several pieces of furniture for stability. It is particularly useful for visiting, when there may not be a suitable chair for the child to use.

Unfortunately chairs which are comfortable for the family may be positively dangerous to the handicapped child, especially if his back is allowed to curve or if insufficient support is given to his neck or shoulder muscles. Physical therapists can advise on the most appropriate support, and their advice should be followed. Handicapped children may not only get into bad habits if they sit in a poor position, they may literally make their handicap worse. If the only chairs available are conventional upholstered armchairs and sofas, the "bean bag" type of chair may be the cheapest alternative. However, very handicapped children may also slump and slip in these, and a child should never be left simply lying unobserved on one for long periods of time. Their great advantage is that they can double as chairs and also as wedges for the child to lie forward on to play on the floor. Children who tend to topple forward are often safer lying instead of sitting to play at floor level, and the prone position on the stomach will often help to strengthen neck and head muscles, must as it helps a normal baby to develop the skills necessary for crawling and mobility. Once again, advice should be sought from the physical therapist, since different handicaps require different support. It is absolutely crucial to avoid perpetuating bad posture, and special furniture and aids, however tempting, should be discussed with a professional familiar with the child before they are introduced into everyday use.

TELEPHONE MODIFICATIONS

It is possible to obtain telephones and adapted equipment in most areas of the country from stores such as Radio Shack and from your local phone company. These telephones have a set of buttons, instead of the conventional dial, and are much easier to operate with poor hand control. They are not designed exclusively for handicapped people, and are available according to supplies.

Southern Bell provides special services for customers with handicaps. Adapted equipment can be obtained at your local AT&T phone center. Modifications for physically handicapped individuals, e.g., Giant Push Button Telephone Adapter and Helping Hand Telephone Holder can be ordered from professional catalogs such as Be OK!

If the disabled caller is deaf or partially hearing, it is possible to rent or purchase an amplifying telephone handset. The amplification is controlled by turning the volume control in the earpiece. If the disabled child can speak only indistinctly, a faint speech amplifier can be fitted to the receiver to raise outgoing calls to normal speech levels. This may be important for children with muscular dystrophy or cerebral palsy, whose speech volume or clarity is reduced by their disability. A control is fitted so that the telephone can be switched back to normal when an able-bodied person wishes to use it.

If somebody is so handicapped that they find difficulty in holding the telephone a headset telephone can be obtained. This is a lightweight headset, plugging into a socket associated with a modified telephone. The telephone is operated by on and off buttons on the headset.

Any person in a wheelchair is likely to find a wallmounted telephone easier to operate than the usual receiver, which is easily knocked onto the floor and has trailing wires. The telephone sales offices are able to advise on this as well as other modifications for the disabled. However, it should be remembered that a telephone is of little use in an emergency if a child cannot use it competently. Practice is needed with making calls, finding numbers, and memorizing emergency procedures. The telephone is an important means of social contact for the disabled, and children should be encouraged to use it within the bounds of economic common sense.

Intercom Systems

Intercom systems are useful to maintain contact between different parts of the home or with neighbors' houses. The majority of systems are battery operated, and consist of two speakers with connecting leads of between 15 and 190 m. The sets can either be switched to "talk" or "listen," or are permanently left on at one end so that any calls or cries are picked up and automatically transmitted. Many of the microphones have limited range and need to be placed close to the handicapped person's bed or chair to be effective.

BEDROOM ADAPTATIONS AND HOISTS

It is worth considering future use carefully, when fitting out a room for a child in a wheelchair. Although bedrooms traditionally occupy the top floors of a house, it may be more sensible (where there is space) to give a handicapped child a groundfloor room. This will save carrying him if he is bedridden, keep him in the mainstream of family life, and greatly facilitate personal freedom in late adolescence when he may wish to go in and out and entertain friends on his own. Although many houses do not have bathrooms on the ground floor that are accessible to wheelchairs, water and drainage are always available near a kitchen. It may be sensible to create a self-contained shower and toilet unit in order to make a self-contained living unit. If the house has a yard, it is frequently possible to extend out into the yard and create, in effect, a one-room apartment with access to the outside. If a house has an awkward elevated front door, with steps and porch, it may be possible to provide access to the road from the room by a side entrance, thus bypassing a narrow or steep entrance.

The bedroom is extremely important to a handicapped person, whether or not it is used as a sitting room. It should be light, bright, and free of unnecessary obstacles in the form of small or free-standing furniture. There should be no small rugs or areas of polished floor.

The type of bed selected depends upon the degree of disability: A child who has limited mobility without a wheelchair may prefer a normal bed; whereas a child who needs to transfer directly to a wheelchair will prefer a bed of equivalent height to his chair. A very handicapped child may be easier to care for on a high hospital-type bed, which will relieve his parents' backs. Since all beds come in standard heights (unless they are hospital-style beds with adjustable bases), it may be necessary to adjust the bed's height with wooden blocks. Bed heights can be increased on some beds by purchasing alternative legs of additional height. As a short-term measure, an extra mattress will give another few inches. If a child is very handicapped and requires constant physical attention, it may be possible to obtain one of the more sophisticated type of beds that can be electrically or manually operated to put the occupant into a sitting position or avoid pressure sores through the constant movement of "rippling" mattresses to generally ease basic care.

Bedclothes are important and should be selected not only for comfort but for ease of laundry and general maintenance. An incontinent child may need clean sheets every day, and there will be a considerable load of washing. It is practical to have a fitted bottom sheet which will not roll up. There are a wide range of machine-washable blankets on the market, but comforters are probably the most comfortable, warm, and economical in terms of bedlinen and bedmaking. They are easily adjusted by handicapped people and are bright and attractive. Many comforters are washable and thus can be used even in cases of incontinence, and they avoid the pressure or restriction of conventional bed-clothes.

If a child suffers from rashes or skin irritations because of incontinence, special sheets can be laid between the rubber under-sheeting and the top sheet. These sheets are made of one-way porous fabric, which filters the urine through, leaving the skin dry and comfortable. A child who is liable to pressure sores may find a medical sheepskin comfortable. Sheepskins can absorb up to their own weight in water before they feel damp, and their deep pile distributes weight over a larger area and avoids localized pressure points. The sheepskins are chemically treated, and can be washed in detergent like wool. Firm cushions on which the child's weight can be distributed can also help in dealing with sores. Some cushions are made following the principle of the beanbag chair. They are filled with polystyrene beads, which shift and adapt to changing body weight. They are also washable.

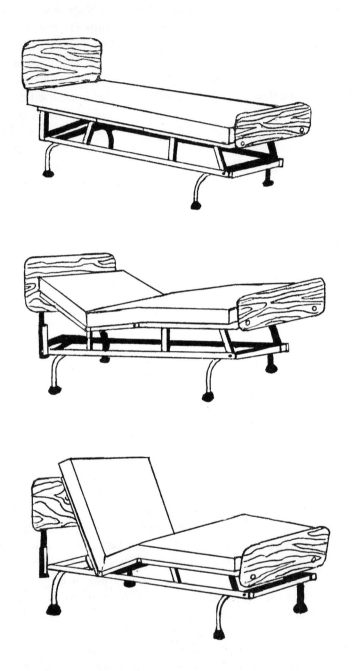

An adjustable bed, manufactured by J. Nesbit-Evans & Co. Ltd., can be moved to three positions.

Clothes should be stored so that they are accessible to a wheelchair. Chests of drawers should be firm and bolted to the wall if there is any risk of them tipping forward. A number of attractive totem pole-type clothes trees are available commercially for nursery use. These are free standing and have various hanging points for clothes, like miniature hat stands. Alternatively, a pole fixed at a suitable height and concealed by a hanging curtain may be the most accessible way of hanging clothes. A vanity unit or dressing table should have a wide work surface, preferably with a large mirror, a light, and drawers close at hand. It is irritating to a wheelchair user to have to keep crossing a room between a variety of pieces of furniture. Since chests of drawers have a habit of suddenly disgorging their drawers and tipping the contents on the floor if pulled too hard, the commercial systems of storage, comprising of wire baskets on runners may be a better method of keeping clothes tidy and close at hand. These can be purchased from most large stores or by mail order, and can be incorporated in a wardrobe fitting. Shoeracks are available in a range of materials and can be hung on the wall, to avoid fumbling on the floor. They are also useful for socks and other odd pieces of clothing which tend to get buried and lost in drawers.

Bed tables are essential. A cantilevered table is the most practical, and should be placed so that it will not be caught by the wheelchair's wheels. Care should always be taken to ensure that bedside tables are stable before they are used for hot drinks or other potential sources of burns or scalds. The larger the table, the more stable it is likely to be. If a child is very clumsy, a thin wooden trim can be glued around the edge to give the protection offered by a ship's table.

A major problem for any paraplegic and many other handicaps is sitting up from a prone position. Some people find a rope ladder or rope attached to the foot of the bed useful to pull against. Many children's toy shops sell rope ladders, but it is relatively simple to manufacture a homemade model from rope and pieces of broom handle or wood knotted in. If the bed has no bed rail, a door handle or similar knob can be screwed into the subframe. This method of pulling up to a sitting position will only work if the child has sufficient movement to bend at the hips in a semireclining position, and if the rope is *securely* fastened.

If direct transfer to the wheelchair is possible, it should be left, with brake on, in a suitable position by the bed. Usually one arm will have to be removed, unless the child prefers to make a front transfer and swivel around. Getting in and out of bed may be very laborious, but most children become very adept, once they have learned the correct technique. It is important that they acquire these techniques, since independence about bedtime and rising will seem very important in adolescent years.

If direct transfer is impossible except by lifting, a hoist may be necessary. Most parents will probably find lifting a young child less trouble than manipulating slings and a winding mechanism, but as the child grows, lifting becomes a considerable strain. There are a large number of hoists available, and advice should be obtained from an occupational therapist about the most appropriate model. The Mecalift (see Appendix B for manufacturer) is a portable hoist that requires a particularly small turning space and is designed for home use. Its chassis height of under four inches enables it to be used with a divan bed. The Hoyer "Travel Lifter Model Hoist" (see Appendix B for manufacturer) can be assembled and dismantled for storage

Portable hoists can be moved around the home. Most have two band slings to support the handicapped person.

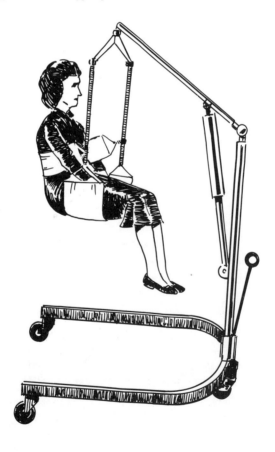

or for carrying in a car trunk. Portable hoists can be used in a number of rooms but require some degree of physical strength in order to maneuver them, particularly in the confined space of the normal family house or apartment. They tend to stick on carpets and cannot be used by the handicapped person alone. Because they are designed to provide movement in restricted space, they are often a compromise between maneuverability and stability. This means that sudden turning or movement, or obstructions, can cause tipping. Hoists need maintenance, and the harness materials in particular should be carefully inspected regularly. However, despite their disadvantages, portable hoists do not take up a great deal of floor space and, with practice, can be used without much difficulty.

A wide range of slings is available for use with different hoists, depending upon particular requirements. Woven nylon slings, which will allow water to drain through, can be used for bathing. The usual method of two band slings is adequate for most handicapped people with some control, but hammock slings support the whole body. Hammock slings are available with headrests, toilet seats, and split legs which supply separate supports for each leg. Choice must depend upon the advice of the occupational therapists.

A range of electrically operated hoists is also available. The hoist runs on a permanent track which is attached to the ceiling joists. An alternative to joist suspension is the fixing of a rolled steel joist into weight-bearing walls. The basic principle behind an overhead hoist is that of the industrial block and tackle: Controls are usually operated by one string for raising and lowering, and another for moving sideways. Since electric hoists are primarily used by severely disabled people, the strings can be knotted or have beads threaded and knotted onto them to provide good grip. Very little strength is needed to operate an electric hoist, and many young people achieve a remarkable degree of independence with one. Hoists can be run out of the bedroom into the bathroom and toilet for complete self-care, but should never be run into bath tubs or shower without the installation of a special isolating transformer.

If a hoist is required for a limited period of time, portable gantries may be used. Gantries resemble a child's swing with a long cross bar. The hoist is suspended on a pulley mechanism and can move sideways between bed and chair. A gantry takes up a considerable amount of floor space, but can be useful during periods of prolonged restricted movement (perhaps following surgery or illness), for which a permanent fixture is not required.

BATHING

Bath and water play are among the most satisfying play experiences for most young children. Physically handicapped children, in particular, can enjoy bathtime for its opportunities for mobility, free movement, and physical sensation. Additionally, of course, anybody who is incontinent will need very regular baths or showers in order to maintain skin hygiene and avoid odor.

Very young handicapped children, whose movements are irregular (with sudden spasms or with very poor muscular tone) may be difficult to manage in a conventional bath. Very often the addition of a nonslip bathmat on the bottom of the tub, or a bath towel similarly placed, will enable a child to be supported by his head and shoulders and kick and splash without any risk of slipping under the water. Large pieces of foam rubber can also be purchased and cut to use as pillows or footrests if there is a real risk of sliding. A special

Special bath seats are available to support the young handicapped child in the bath.

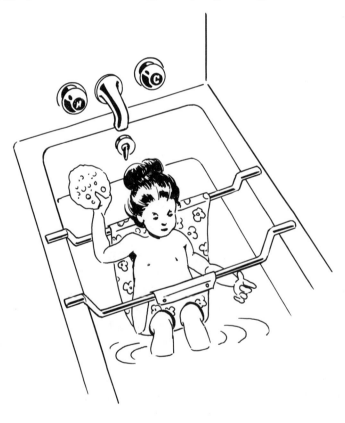

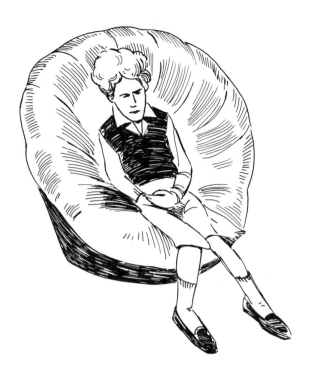

The "Suzy chair is an inflatable chair resembling a shell.
It can be used in the bath or in the house.

bath seat can be purchased made of soft plastic, with leg holes and
back support, which is hooked across the bath rather like a soap
rack. The advantage of a seat is that the water level can be increased
and the child can freely kick and splash with his hands and feet. The
mother is also freed from maintaining balance with one hand and
soaping and washing with the other. Some mothers have also experimented quite successfully with a plastic laundry basket in the bath
(the water filtering through the holes, and the rounded edges offering
quite good support to a small child). If soaping is a problem—since
there is nothing more slippery than a soapy and wriggling toddler—
there are a number of bubble baths and baby-care bath liquids that
can be added directly to the bath water. These do not require rinsing
and have the added advantage of providing bubbles for amusement.
However, some children may have specially sensitive skins and care
should be taken not to overdo liquid soaps if they irritate the skin.

As a child gets bigger, bathtime becomes more problematic. Not
only does the child want a degree of independence (and perhaps
privacy), but he is also heavier, and there is a greater risk of slipping
or falling. Many handicapped children can transfer themselves from

their wheelchair to a bath board or bath seat across the end of the bath. If there is a grab rail on the wall above the bath, they can then swing safely down into the water. Needless to say, nonslip bathmats are essential, unless the tub is one of the newer fiberglass models with a textured base to prevent slipping. Tubs will, in any event, be safer if the faucets are set on the corner, and if there are handles incorporated in the sides of the tub.

Tubs and Basins

All bathrooms used by handicapped people should have nonslip floors. Unpolished textured vinyl or cork tiles are inexpensive and easy to maintain. It is also sensible to have a nonslip absorbent mat on the floor to prevent pools of water from collecting and making dangerous slippery areas. Bathrooms should be warm (a handicapped adolescent bathing himself may take twice as long undressing and dressing as an able-bodied child. Wall-mounted radiators or electric heaters (above eye level) are safest. Oil heaters and any form of portable electric heater or hair dryer should *never* be used in a bathroom, however tempting and economical they may appear to be.

If you are modifying or building a bathroom, it is sensible to take a careful look at available fittings. A handicapped child is part of the family, and the main bathroom must meet *all* the family's needs. But certain simple considerations may save time and energy and actually make bathtime a more comfortable procedure. Because many handicapped children are able to get themselves into the bath via a bath seat or sliding board, it is sensible (if possible) to create the maximum floor space for maneuvering the wheelchair.

Many modern bathtubs are very low. This is convenient for anyone stepping in, but difficult and dangerous for a direct transfer from a wheelchair. Since the wheelchair's average height is about 480 mm (about 19 in.), the bathtub should be a similar height. Bathtubs also vary in depth: Some are shallow, some deep; some are shorter than others. Although a short bathtub is primarily intended for awkward installation in a small space, it may be useful for a handicapped person because there is less risk of slipping under the water in a prone position. Shallow bathtubs are also safer and are much easier for a helper, if lifting is involved. Sunken bathtubs will not be within the budget of most families, but can have advantages if an older child can get out of his wheelchair onto the floor and then slide into the bathtub. They are, however, extremely dangerous if the floor is slippery and if there is little space to turn the wheelchair. The new bathtubs with textured and squared-off bases are much safer, because of the diminished risk of slipping. However, nonslip bathmats can be purchased at any large store and can be used in any tub. Nonslip bathmats are usually plastic, with suction cups on one side to grip the tub. They should not be left lying in the water at the bottom of the bathtub, because they are liable to become slimy and slippery, especially if the faucets tend to drip. The mat should be removed after use and put on one side to dry. Bathtubs made of plastic or fiberglass have the added advantage of being slightly softer and warmer to touch, and they mean less risk of injury in a fall, but they are also more vulnerable to rough treatment.

Getting into the Bath

Rails and hand grips need to be strong and correctly placed. A handicapped person is likely to put more weight on an appliance than an able-bodied person (who is likely to use rails simply for balance). Although rails built into a bathtub are useful, they are usually too low to help on the last stages of getting out. If a rail is too close to the wall, it is impossible to get a hand around it. If it is made of rough or slippery metal, it may damage the hands, or be dangerous when wet. This is particularly important if the rail is fitted on a slant or vertically. Handrails can also be purchased or made to clamp onto the side of the bathtub. They should be fitted at the faucet end of the bathtub to give maximum space—and if the bathtub is not metal, protection will be needed for the clamps to avoid damaging the surface.

Handrails can be purchased to clamp onto the side of the bathtub.

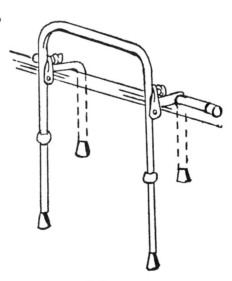

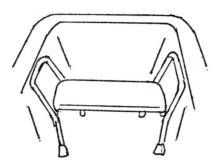

Bath seats help a handicapped child to get in and out of the bathtub.

The conventional bath stool, with four sturdy legs and a nonslip cork seat, may offer a convenient halfway point between wheelchair and tub. However, most people with little use of their legs prefer a bath board. Bath boards can be bought or made, but they need to fit the bath and to be stable. They can be covered with plastic for easy movement or with cork if a warm or stable surface is required. Since a paraplegic can obviously not very easily transfer from a board that is 19 in. high to the bottom of the tub in one movement, a bath seat may be useful. These can be removed or used as a base for washing. But care should be taken in purchasing a bath seat for a fiberglass tub, because fiberglass "gives" and eventually may be damaged by the pressure of the hard seat rims. Alternative seats can be purchased which hook over the side of the bathtub.

Although some very severely handicapped children can (with the very considerable strength of unaffected arms) swing themselves in and out of a bathtub with minimal problem, it is prudent never to let a child bathe without an adult in easy reach. Accidents do happen, and while independence is the end in view, it is better to avoid any risk of a sudden fall.

Severely handicapped children may need special consideration over bathing routines. Bath seats and bath boards presuppose good use of arm and shoulder muscles, but some children will never achieve this degree of independence, and their parents will need much more assistance with bathtime routines. Though many parents feel, when their children are little, that they can cope with bathtime by conventional methods and that the special aids and appliances now available are too complicated to contemplate, children grow bigger, parents get older. There is the increased risk of parents hurting their own backs by lifting and carrying. It is worth considering some of the recent developments while a child is still young and light enough to help relatively easily through the trial and error period before techniques are fully mastered.

Since many families will not have new bathtubs or specially built bathrooms, they will have to adapt existing facilities. A useful aid to counteract the problems of a very deep bath and a heavy child is the *bath shell* (see diagram). This is molded from rigid plastic and fits over the bath. It is filled from faucets on the existing bathtub. Different shapes allow for bathing in the prone position (particularly useful for hair washing and quite safe as the water level is very low) and for bathing in a semisitting position. The "bath shape" can easily be removed and stored upright when not in use. It can, *in extremis,* travel on vacation on a car roof rack when bath facilities are likely to be difficult. Another method of creating a more shallow bath (and avoiding lifting in and out) is an inflated air bed in the base of the tub or a bath cushion. Bath cushions are filled with water like a water bed, and as they fill, they reduce the depth of the bath. They can be filled to a level comparable with the top of the bath and then deflated gradually with the bather in situ. A useful control for a severely handicapped child is the *Suzy* inflatable chair. Inflated, it forms a shell shape which can be securely wedged into the bath and will hold the child in a relaxed sitting position. It can also be used as a playroom chair. A variety of other bath seats are available, but many are difficult to lift a large or very handicapped child in and out of.

There are a number of hoists on the market, and it is vital that a family has professional advice on suitability and availability, and that they are *shown* how to use one. Most hoists are simple to use, but require a knack if slipping and jolting are to be avoided. Some parents find it helpful to practice with an able-bodied member of the

The bath shell is a shallow bath inserted into a conventional bathtub to enable handicapped people to be bathed safely and with minimum effort. It can be filled from the bathtub faucets and emptied through its own plug. It is manufactured by Sunflower Bathing Aids.

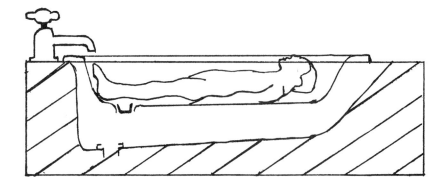

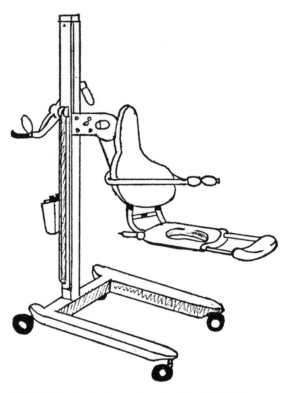

The "Droitwich Bathing System" combines the "Spa Bath Lift"
with direct chair-to-bath transfer.

family, since positioning of slings and so forth is very important for
comfort and safety.

Hoists for use in the bathroom may either be operated on an
electric track (possibly running from the bedroom down the corridor for a very severely handicapped person), or be fitted into a
socket in the floor, or be mobile (and usable in other rooms in the
house). Floor or ceiling installations clearly require expert opinion
on the suitability of joists and the availability of sufficient space. A
permanent hoist will take up a good deal of room in a small bathroom, but in general the permanently fixed hoists are easier to
operate than the mobile ones, which must be manually pumped up
and down and which (for obviously safety reasons) have to counteract their mobility with weight for stability. Although most hoists
hold the child in two or three slings, some are specially designed for
bathroom use with a seat shaped like a toilet seat and made of rigid
plasic. This seat goes right into the bath, and if there is no attendant,
can be used during the bath and then manually returned to storage

position. The child can be dried and dressed sitting in the seat and then be transferred directly to the wheelchair.

Showers

As a severely handicapped child gets older, the problems of bathing (even with a hoist) may assume alarming proportions. It may also be quite impossible to give the child any degree of privacy because of the need for an adult to oversee the whole bathing process. When bathing is difficult, the answer may be a shower. If the family is large, this can have the added advantage that a shower is quite easily fitted into a bedroom, and the bathroom can then be released for other members of the family at "peak times." Obviously a child in a wheelchair cannot easily use the conventional shower cabinet. However, showers can easily be set into a tiled area (with central drain, as so often seen in Mediterranean countries) which is on a level (apart from a slight downward slope) with the rest of the room. The child can then either transfer directly from his wheelchair onto a bench-type seat at the side of the shower, or onto a special shower seat (rather like a plastic toilet seat) which will let the water run through. Mobile shower chairs can be obtained for use in both shower and bathroom. The child can transfer in his own room and propel it along with a cane or with a foot. Showers used in this way must have thermostatic control; the tiles need to be nonslip, and the room's

Special shower seats enable a child to use a shower independently.

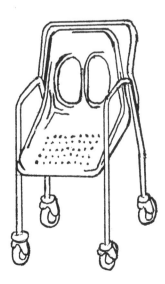

167

other floor covering impervious to the occasional splash. Cord or cork floor coverings are particularly suitable to wheelchair rooms.

Showers can offer enormous advantages to those children whose dependency needs are greatest—such as the more severely affected spina bifida children and paraplegics. They are more hygienic than baths for the incontinent; they avoid the basic problem of transfer into the bathtub and (more problematically) getting out of the bathtub and back into a wheelchair. They are space saving and economical in terms of installation and hot water supply. They additionally permit children in wheelchairs to enjoy a greater degree of privacy. Many children, particularly in early adolescence, are acutely aware of their disabilities, of any abnormalities in their bodies, and, in particular, of the social stigma of incontinence—urinary devices, incontinence pads, or diapers. In a busy family bathroom, where it may be almost impossible to shut the door if a wheelchair and portable hoist are wheeled in, the whole family may be in and out during the hour or so of "self-care" that most spina bifida children have to work through each evening. It is scarcely surprising, in these circumstances, that handicapped children grow up feeling different; that their bodies are somehow public property, belonging not to themselves but to the doctors who so constantly examine and consider them, *and* to the family who have to support an extensive program of self-care.

Washbasins

Any wheelchair user will find a wall-hung basin (preferably set into a vanity unit type of top) easiest to use for washing, attention to hair and teeth, and general cosmetic activities. If it is not possible to alter an existing pedestal-type basin in the bathroom, it may be possible to provide a suitable basin in the bedroom. A large mirror will help with difficult buttons, combing of hair, and so forth for a child with poor hand control. Many faucet handles are difficult for weak fingers to operate, and these can be exchanged for short levers that can easily be operated with an elbow or a finger. If the basin area is also a dressing table (with suitable working surface), much time and effort on self-care will be saved.

Many handicapped people find hair and teeth difficult to attend to. Lengthening hairbrush handles with pieces of stiff rubber or plastic tubing may help. Also, a length of broom handle can have a hole bored at an appropriate point to hold a comb. If a child has virtually no hand control, the brush can be attached to a rigid piece of wood and fastened to a chair. By sitting in the chair and moving his or her head, the child can achieve some measure of control. Some children find the traditional men's hairbrushes (flat with a handle across the back of the brush) easy to use.

Toothbrushes can be lengthened in the same way as hairbrushes. Alternatively, electric toothbrushes may prove a solution to the problem, since minimum pressure is required to use them.

Hairwashing is a major problem for many parents. If the child can lie back in the bath (perhaps with neck supported on a foam wedge), it may be easiest to wash the hair there. A hose attached to the faucet or shower will help with rinsing. Mothercare sells a face-guard for young children which fits around the face like a halo and keeps soapy water out of the eyes. Older children may find that the use of a plastic sun visor or swimming goggles performs the same function. If it is not possible for an older child to lean forward and if there is no shower, it may be easier to back the wheelchair up to a suitable table and wash the hair backwards in a basin. A special attachment can be purchased to fit onto a basin or sink by suction cups, so that hair can be washed backwards. Shampoo trays on adjustable stands as used by hairdressers, can also be used in the home. Alternatively, a number of nursing-aid plastic bowls have hose attachments for emptying water into a bucket, and can be used for children who are bed-bound for any reason.

Hair can be blow-dried or dried with a hood drier. An adolescent girl may be very anxious to have a hair style in keeping with her age group, and cutting, perming, and setting may prove to be a problem. However, many wheelchairs can quite conveniently be wheeled up to the basin in a hairdressers, provided that the chairs usually used can be moved and that advance enquiries have been made about height of basins and dryers. Many local papers also contain advertisements by hairdressers prepared to visit the house. And if all this is impossible, family experimentation with heated rollers, blow drying, and electric curling irons may be the answer. Appearances *do* matter—and mothers may have to discipline themselves and be prepared to help achieve a hair style even if they consider it eminently unsuitable!

General washing aids can usually be purchased from drugstores or made at home. There is a wide range of washing mittens (much more convenient than washcloths when hand control is weak), soaps on cords (which can be secured to faucets), and other bathing aids which make self-care easier. If a child has poor hand control, a piece of soap can be inserted into one sponge for washing, and another sponge used for rinsing. Alternatively, the wide range of baby detergents which can be poured into water and do not need rinsing eliminate the need for soap altogether. Wherever possible, it is preferable to use "normal" bathing aids and to modify as little as possible—both for future practicality and for the child's own self-image.

GOING TO THE TOILET

The majority of wheelchair children will be able to manage toilet routines for themselves—if they can only get proper access. In many homes, the traditional placing of the commode on a narrow wall directly facing an inward-opening door makes access virtually impossible for a wheelchair. If it is not possible to create a larger bathroom elsewhere in the house, an alternative may be to relocate the commode on a side wall against the farthest corner of the room—wheelchair users normally find side access easiest. An inward-opening door can either be reversed to open outward, or a sliding or folding door can be installed in its place.

As a child gets larger, and assistance is more burdensome for parents or helper, advice should be obtained from a physical therapist about the easiest way to get onto the toilet. A suitably

Plastic toilet seats can be purchased to raise the height of the toilet bowl. They are also useful for vacations and trips.

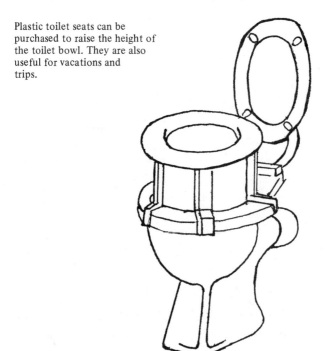

positioned hand rail "bell-pull" suspended from the ceiling will enable many children to pull themselves upright and transfer sideways to the toilet. A sliding board may be used, or, alternatively, the seat can be cut into a bench-type fitting extending across a wider area. These "pew"-type toilet fittings, which are hinged to the wall for lifting and cleaning, were popular in Victorian bathrooms. They are convenient today in giving a wide safe area for maneuvering and for supporting body weight by the arms and hands. Side maneuvers will not normally be possible unless the toilet seat is approximately the same height as the wheelchair. Since 19 in. is higher than the average modern bathroom fitting (which is usually 14 to 16 in. high), various adjustments may need to be made. If a wooden bench seat is fitted, this can incorporate the additional thickness. Otherwise the toilet bowl can be lifted up on a fireclay or wooden frame, or alternatively, a variety of special plastic toilet seats can be purchased to clip onto the bowl. A portable seat can also be taken on visits and trips.

A low toilet may cause difficulties for a handicapped person by catching their back and arms. Toilet frames can be built around the commode to give support. They are particularly useful for disabled people who need to push, rather than pull, themselves up; they also offer useful support in adjusting clothes, but will only be really practical for the more able-bodied wheelchair users. If it is quite impossible to maneuver a wheelchair in the available space to effect a side transfer, it may be worth acquiring a toilet chair. This is a chair on wheels, with a soft plastic or rubber toilet seat replacing the conventional hard chair base. Some can also be used in showers. The chair must be provided in a suitable size to "ride over" the toilet, and can either be pushed or "punted" along by its occupant pushing along the wall with a hand, or using one foot or a cane along the ground. If space is really crowded, this strategy may be preferable to endeavoring to turn a wheelchair and risk damaging equipment and paint, and possibly falling.

Many severely disabled people have great difficulty in cleaning themselves after visits to the toilet. This is particularly true where hand control or balance is weak. Soft paper is easier to use than hard paper. Packets of paper tissues conveniently placed on an adjacent wall are easier to manipulate than the conventional toilet rolls. Some toilet seats are horseshoe shaped, with a front opening, which also makes cleaning easier. Alternatively, it may be possible to purchase a special lavatory that combines lavatory, bidet, and warm air drying operated from an electric switch. This would be particularly useful

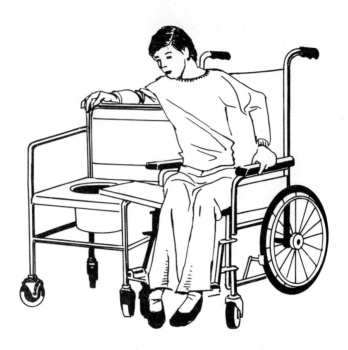

A sliding board can be used to direct transfer between the wheelchair and toilet or commode chair.

for people in need of regular douching or washing because of incontinence. Its cost, though, will put it outside the price bracket of most families. The normal low bidet is of little use to most wheelchair users, because of access. But a portable plastic bidet can be purchased which can be filled by a hose from a faucet or jug. It has a small plug for emptying directly into the toilet and may be preferable to bed washes for an incontinent child.

Despite the increasing sophistication of plastic pants, incontinence aids, and deodorants, it should never be forgotten that handicapped children cannot afford the additional indignity of *smelling*. Stale urine quickly produces an unpleasant ammoniac smell, whether on the baby who needs a diaper change or the able-bodied child who regularly wets his bed and is allowed to go to school unwashed. In either case, the family of the child may be so accustomed to the odor that they regard it as part of their normal environment. Other people will not be so generous, and where incontinence appliances are worn, cleanliness should be scrupulous and part of a daily routine. In the case of incontinence, a daily shower or bath may be quite insufficient.

Managing Clothes

The art of safely lifting yourself on and off the commode is not the only problem which disabled children will have to master. Management of clothing may be a major problem—and one which the able-bodied rarely consider. A child in a wheelchair with strong arms may not have any great problem in this area, but a general separation of clothes into top and bottom halves will facilitate adjustments. Girls' skirts can be wraparounds, fastening with velcro, and boys' trousers can be similarly adjusted with velcro.

DOMESTIC SKILLS

Kitchen sense is vital for a disabled child. Since future independence will depend to a large extent upon the child's ability to care for himself, a survival kit of basic domestic skills is essential. Although it is important never to "think handicapped," it is equally necessary to encourage a child in a wheelchair to think realistically about his abilities. Some children are so overprotected at home and school that they never have a real opportunity to try new projects or to come to terms with their own disability. They may, indeed, have a totally unrealistic view of what they should do. If our overall aim is independence compatible with the degree of disability, children will have to acquire some skills which may seem difficult and tedious, some of which will never fully be mastered. But it is infinitely better to learn these in childhood than to come to grief in independent housing or in marriage as an adult. Many able-bodied children, of course, never acquire more than minimal domestic skills; and they manage their lives quite competently. But they can, of course, afford to fail. A child who has spent a good deal of time in a residential unit may, in particular, fail to realize just how much work goes into preparing and cleaning up after a meal. He may never have really thought about the time-consuming processes of laundry and mending. It is better to learn the problems of domestic routines when young.

The Kitchen

If a family has been able to build or modify its house so that the kitchen is adapted to suit a wheelchair, access and working space will not be a problem. But most families with a handicapped child will not have a specially-built kitchen. Indeed, if they had, the worktops would probably not be the correct height for the rest of the family. For obvious reasons, wheelchair users need lower work surfaces, and there is a basic problem of access and safety in using a kitchen that is not made to measure.

Even if a kitchen cannot be properly modified, certain criteria can perhaps be met which will make the kitchen environment safer and more attractive for the whole family. Split-level stoves have obvious advantages for handicapped people. A built-in oven with a door which opens downward offers good physical and visual access to a wheelchair user. Most electric ovens (and a few gas ones) have interior glass doors which mean that cooking can be observed without repeated opening and shutting of the oven door. The new ceramic stoves, which do not have raised burners, offer an additional safety component, since pans will not slip and spill when being moved on and off the heat. Controls for many cabinet units are set at the side or back of the unit. This is normally a useful safety precaution where there are small children around. But a handicapped child, seated at a lower level, may risk burns or scalds if he has to reach a hand over the heat surface and pans to adjust controls. It is safer to set them at the side or near the front of the cabinet unit.

Because of the dangers of scalds or burns, a work surface continuous to the sink is very necessary. Sinks can be recessed directly into the work surface without a draining board, to give a completely flat track between heat surface or oven and water. The traditional draining board is not absolutely necessary, and if a double sink is installed, its place can be taken by a plastic rack in the second sink. If it is not possible to alter an existing kitchen, the child may need to wash up and use water in a bowl on a table.

The dangers of hot water should not be minimized, particularly for children wth paraplegia or spina bifida who have little or no feeling in their lower limbs. These children should therefore wear a suitable protective apron. A plastic or vinyl apron can be backed with padding made from dishcloths or old woolen material. This can be held in place with a material backing which can be glued to the top apron. Needless to say, no child should be allowed to carry kettles or pans of boiling water.

Electric outlets in a kitchen for handicapped people should be at work-surface height, so that toasters and electric coffee pots do not have wires trailing on the floor. There is a very real risk of injury if a wheelchair wheel or crutch catches a wire and a piece of electric apparatus is pulled off a table or cupboard top. For safety reasons, electric equipment with automatic timing devices is preferable to equipment requiring more control. Electric toasters and coffee pots are all available with cutoff switches or timers, and these can save bad accidents.

Since a clumsy child is much more likely to spill fat or fail to adjust a burner in time, a small fire extinguisher should be part of every kitchen. Most people set a pan on fire at least once in a lifetime, and disabled people will need immediate tools at hand to avert disaster.

Storage and cupboards may present problems in any kitchen. Many modern kitchens offer storage facilities at wall as well as at floor level. If a handicapped child is to share the kitchen, basic china and foodstuffs should be kept in lower cupboards. Reaching upwards is dangerous, especially if heavy jars or pieces of china are involved. Many kitchen units now have shelves on runners, sometimes with optional basket fittings, which pull right out. Other shelves rotate, so that easy access is available to all parts. These internal fittings make life much easier for a handicapped person. It is very difficult to reach to the back of a deep cupboard—and potentially dangerous, since jars or cans are easily dislodged to fall and break on the floor. Small jars of spice and flavorings can be stored in narrow shelves with protective bars on the inside of cupboard doors. If catches are difficult to open, magnetic catches can be substituted. These are easily operated with minimum effort.

There is a wide range of electrical equipment to simplify day-to-day cooking. The electric toaster and kettle are probably in most kitchens. But a good food mixer can be invaluable when hand control is poor and mixing and beating prove difficult. Some children will find the large mixers difficult to manage, since some effort is needed to insert and remove the mixing bowl. But there is a wide range of hand mixers which can be used in a pan or saucepan according to need. Some have special blades so that there is no risk of injury to fingers.

The type of saucepan used will to a large extent depend upon the kind of stove available. Some children will find heavy saucepans more stable and less easy to tip. If there is a continuous work surface between the burners and the sink, pans can be slid along, rather than lifted, and water tipped out when the pan is in the sink. But some children will find weight difficult to manage and will prefer lightweight pans. Nonstick pans are much easier for cleaning and for stirring and blending. A number of kitchenware sets now include a saucepan that has two handles and can be used as a saucepan on the stove or a casserole in the oven. The two handles may make this much more maneuverable than a single-handed saucepan. Oven roasts can also be cooked in the plastic roasting bags (which have the advantage of being see-through), or in kitchen foil to avoid unnecessary cleaning of the oven. Since economy is regrettably likely to be a major factor in a handicapped person's adult life, experimentation with cooking vegetables in casseroles in the oven with a roast will save fuel and unnecessary handling of pans of hot water.

For safety considerations, a suitable floor should be chosen which is nonslip and easy to clean. Some vinyl floors are very slippery when wet, and care should be taken to choose a suitable material. Since wheelchairs will almost certainly make dirty marks on a floor which is likely to receive spills, an easy-to-clean surface is also sensible. It is better to avoid rugs or mats which can get dangerously entwined with wheelchairs. Lighting is very important, particularly if a child in a wheelchair is using work surfaces that are high. Strip lighting can be installed under wall cupboards and gives a good diffused light.

The Kitchen as an Aid to Independence

Many mothers feel exceedingly irritated by their normal children's efforts in the kitchen. It may seem to be inviting even more irritation to encourage a handicapped child to undertake tasks which will produce mess and consume time. But the overall aim is not only to offer enjoyment, but, even more important, to produce, eventual capability to run a home. If a handicapped person marries, which the increased availability of modified housing makes more probable, he or she will in all probability marry someone else with a handicap. (This is largely because social opportunities are greater to meet people with similar problems, but it may also be because two handicapped people will have a great deal of mutual understanding of their physical problems and needs.) In this case, it is vital that the man and woman have basic skills sufficient to care for themselves and each other. Even if a handicapped man or woman acquires an able-bodied partner, the situation remains acute, because he or she will wish to be as normal as possible, however caring the partner. The handicapped will be anxious to establish himself or herself as a member of a normal world and to take a full part in the organization of the home.

Independence in the domestic setting will mean different things for different people. It will mean a realistic appraisal of everything that is involved in running a home, from budgeting and shopping to cooking a meal and washing up, and it may mean a degree of "planned dependence" when the child knows that he cannot complete a task without help. For this reason, it is not a disaster if a child sticks mainly to convenience foods. If a family normally eats frozen foods and prefers fish sticks to anything else anyway, then the food prepared will be within this range; and many very handicapped people will be able to prepare very simple meats using frozen or canned ingredients. Fresh meat and vegetables require more skill, though it is of course essential that knowledge of basic cooking should be acquired if possible. No one wants to live on baked beans all the time, and food can have a social significance for the disabled which it perhaps now lacks for the able-bodied.

Whatever type of food is cooked, care should be taken to talk about the reasons for selecting certain foods, about the need to eat fresh fruit, vegetables, and meat. Many fresh vegetables can be cooked very simply by a handicapped person: Potatoes can be baked in jackets, and root vegetables can be casseroled in the oven rather than in a heavy pan on the stove. Meat can be purchased chopped for cooking, and casseroles are easy to make and handle if the oven is side-opening. Since (unfortunately) income is small for most disabled people, thought should be given to budgeting and low-cost food. But the overall aim should be to ensure that a meal will offer maximum variety and nutritional value with minimum effort.

Cooking as Play

Cooking can be very useful in encouraging a child with poor hand control to use his hands and exercise his muscles. Bread making, with kneading and pulling, is usually popular and gives good results however roughly the dough is handled! Cakes require mixing and whisking, and icing requires coordination of eye and fingers. Here, cake mixes and other packets should not be despised: creaming butter and sugar may take too long or be too hard for a very handicapped child. The cake mix will produce a quick and palatable result with less effort. Young children will also usually enjoy making pastry and cutting out cookie shapes. Pastry can be tinted with vegetable dyes, and gingerbread figures and other fancy cutters can make pretty cookies.

There is a wide range of children's cook books on the market, which give clear visual instructions for a variety of simple dishes. Cooking is an activity dear to all children, and it can help attract unhandicapped children in the neighborhood. Cooking as well as eating can be social affairs, and the mother who lets her kitchen be taken over by children on a rainy afternoon will ensure a good deal of popularity for herself and her child! If a number of children are using the kitchen, it is usually safer to put them at a table. The traditional hard-wood kitchen table has made a comeback and offers an admirable stable surface for pastry making, cutting, and other domestic activities. It is relevant to reflect that cooking is an excellent communal activity for the shy child, and is well worth the mess afterwards!

SMALL AIDS AROUND THE HOME

People in wheelchairs may find life easier if they use some of the small aids and adaptations which can be easily made at home or purchased. There are a number of reaching and picking-up devices for reaching into cupboards and shelves and on to for picking up from the floor. These can also be used for operating light switches, turning on heaters, or pulling the curtains shut. Picking-up devices usually fall into three main kinds. Some resemble large scissors; others are like extending tongs, and some are lever-operated sticks, with a "jaw" at the end for picking things up. The type of device used will depend on the length of reach required and the strength of the hand muscles. Some are stiffer than others, and it is often useful to experiment with several models. Some of the longer devices are very useful for long-distance reaching (for pulling curtains or reaching high shelves) but are obviously heavy. They can therefore be dangerous if hand control is too weak to use them properly and, if allowed to fall, may break ornaments or damage decorations.

Some children find the pick-up sticks very difficult to manipulate and prefer the long-handled dustpans, which can be purchased in any large store. These can be used as scoops to pick up toys from the floor. One child found a toy fishing net, with its cane handle suitably bound with rubber to prevent injuries, very satisfactory. Most reaching devices are designed for adult people and may therefore be awkward for a small child. Even if they are easily maneuvered, care should be taken when reaching upward. Heavy objects can easily slip if pulled forward and downward from shelves, and it is safer to store the child's possessions and toys at or below waist level if possible.

Children who can walk a little with aids may find handrails very useful. Handrails should be placed in accordance with the occupational therapist's or physical therapist's suggestions. Needless to say, they should be absolutely secure; handicapped children are likely to put heavy stress on them, and they should be carefully tested. Often small handrails or grips are useful; a wide range of metal and wooden handles are available at do-it-yourself shops and can provide a useful balance at doors or at turns in the corridor. Longer handrails will also help save the decorations, since the child can run his hand along them rather than along the paint or paper.

Many gadgets are really no more than minor adjustments to normal household equipment. Curtains are much easier to pull if they are operated by a cord. This also prolongs their life and cleanliness. Doors are often a problem for the handicapped, and their opening and shutting can be eased by roller catches, which allow the door to be moved by pressure against it, or by lever handles. The traditional knobs are very difficult to turn, if hand control is poor.

If an older handicapped child is considering how he may eventually cope with a home alone—or if it is decided that *all* the family must share the household chores—there are many ways of making housework easier. Most stores now sell dusting mittens and these can also be made cheaply at home, and can be used for spreading polish or cleaner and for polishing. If they have ties, they can be fastened to the wheelchair to avoid dropping. Household cleansers are almost all available in aerosol form. Whatever one feels about polluting the atmosphere with aerosols, they have enormous advantages in providing instant and controllable quantities of cleaner or polish. Their shape also makes them simple to carry in a bag attached to the wheelchair, or to put into a shoerack which can hang at an appropriate place. Feather dusters are still available (or a traditional dish mop can be lengthened with a length of rubber tubing) for dusting. Vacuum cleaners can be used from a wheelchair, but their wires tend to catch in the wheels, and they are heavy to control. A more suitable appliance may be one of the new lightweight carpet sweepers. Many of these are now adjusted to operate on both hard and carpeted floors, and have brush attachments to work around corners. If the child is short or small, it is worth choosing one of the carpet sweepers with retractable or slotted handles. A piece of handle can then be removed so that the sweeper is the right height for the child, and there is no risk of pokes in the face or body.

Laundry is important also, although most families have a washing machine or go to a laundromat. Much of the hard work can be taken out of hand washing by buying suitable clothes, always washing them before they are really dirty and soaking before washing. Bleaches are very effective, particularly with soiled linen or whites which are soaked before washing. However, care should be taken that they are properly rinsed out of clothes and that they do not cause rashes or other skin irritation. Pure detergents may be preferable if the washed clothes are uncomfortable.

Since so many clothes are drip-dry, ironing may not seem very important. But ironing is still necessary for creases in trousers or best clothes, and it is sensible to get children started young! Most ironing boards are adjustable to a range of heights; and some kitchens have pullout ironing boards which are particularly safe because the problem of the legs is removed. Ironholders can be purchased which hold the iron (hot or cold) in a vertical position. These remove the risk of trailing wires and can be fastened onto walls or cupboards. Children with paraplegia or poor sensation in their limbs need to be careful when handling anything hot and should be encouraged to develop a regular routine when using any electrical appliances.

If mending is necessary, self-threading needles or threaders can be purchased from any sewing shop or department. If poor hand control makes sewing quite impossible, the various iron-on tapes can be experimented with. Scissors are available for left- or right-hand cutting, and Stirex scissors have a spring that enables them to be operated like tongs by pressing the fingers inward. Electric scissors are also available, though they clearly need care and observation when first used. It is worth encouraging an interest in sewing, since many children with physical handicaps will have problems in finding suitable clothes. If the boy or girl can alter, adapt, or make his or her own clothes, a good deal of money can be saved as well as an interesting hobby gained.

9

Special Education: The Physically Handicapped Child

Under the terms of Public Law 94-142, school districts are empowered to provide special facilities for handicapped children from the age of two. However, despite good intentions, many parts of the country still lack basic facilities for very young handicapped children, and the parent of a child in a wheelchair may encounter the school authorities only when their child reaches the age of five.

The basic conflict for parents selecting a first school will probably be the question of whether to choose segregated education or integrated education. Many education authorities place their major teaching resources for handicapped children firmly in the special school. Speech therapy, physical therapy, and trained teachers are more likely to be found in the special school setting where equipment is better and classes smaller. The general commitment of educationalists and the government is toward full participation by the handicapped in the community, but there are at present simply not the resources in the ordinary schools to back up teachers in providing handicapped children with all they need. Integration without positive discrimination could be disastrous for children already heavily penalized in the quest for a good education.

In fact, current usage of the terms *integration* and *segregation* tends to confuse the issue, since both terms cover a multitude of possible alternatives. Handicapped children are not necessarily integrated simply by being slotted into classrooms in a normal school. For one thing, they will always need extra provisions, such as sensitive and consistent help with toileting, participation in physical activities, and perhaps supervision in the rough and tumble of the corridor or classroom. If integration is a special class in a normal school, there may be barriers between the children and the other pupils. Not only will special resources be needed in the normal school (where larger classes additionally compound the extra time which a physically handicapped child requires for very ordinary activities), but the staff themselves must avoid overindulgent or protective attitudes to the child. A spina bifida boy in one normal school spent the whole time during the physical education exercises sitting in his wheelchair. No one has told his teacher that he could perfectly and easily move about on the floor or on a simple apparatus where his arms could compensate for his paralyzed legs. She assumed that he was at risk of injury; he assumed that he was forbidden from participating. In a special school, he would have had extensive opportunities for hydrotherapy, physical therapy, and regular exercise out of his chair. In the normal school, despite having an aide in addition to the teacher, the staff lacked the specific information necessary to meet his needs. He was therefore exceedingly isolated in a normal school. On the other hand, another spina bifida child (a twelve-year-old girl) attended a comprehensive school with a number of other physically handicapped children. The school was supported by visiting special advisers and by a full-time aide who had been trained in working with handicapped children. The teacher was committed to the idea of integration. The school offered a wide range of subjects and, with its larger pupil intake, was a stimulating and lively environment for the handicapped girl. She was therefore able to be fully integrated and well adjusted, despite a major physical handicap.

In considering the question of "special" versus "normal," it is therefore crucial to separate long-term objectives from short-term needs. Most educationists and parents are now committed in the long term to the social necessity of a greater degree of integration—the nineteenth century notion of the "cripple" as an object of charity isolated from the rest of the world is fortunately dead. But parents now find that the twin objectives of wishing to achieve a normal life style for their child and, at the same time, to enable him to acquire maximum skills for his development, are not easily reconcilable. In effect, parents have to look at local facilities and make decisions for themselves. The situation within school districts with well-established systems of special education, for instance, are very different from that in other districts with few physical resources in the form of buildings, but with more flexible services in terms of teachers and special classes attached to normal schools.

Additionally, attitudes of individual school principals vary in different areas—and their goodwill is crucial for successful integration.

Social adaptation and independence, which are integral parts of education, do not necessarily automatically "happen" in an integrated atmosphere. If the child is smothered with help and affection at home—or if he is neglected in a variety of subtle ways—he may need a good deal of encouragement to act on his own initiative. The special school, with its pool of resources, is uniquely equipped to help handicapped children realize that they *can* become achievers.

FEDERAL LEGISLATION

Two federal laws—P.L. (Public Law) 94-142 (the Education for All Handicapped Children Act of 1975) and P.L. 93-112 (the Rehabilitation Act of 1973) have applied relevant court rulings to handicapped children in the schools.

P.L. 93-112 (Section 504) states that no handicapped person can be denied benefits because of his handicap in any program or activity receiving federal government assistance that is, public schools.

P.L. 94-142 requires that all handicapped individuals from birth to twenty-one years of age receive equal educational opportunities and a free appropriate public education (f.a.p.e.). The six major sections of this law are (1) zero reject, (2) nondiscriminatory evaluation, (3) individualized and appropriate education, (4) least restrictive environment, (5) procedural due process, and (6) parent participation.

Zero Reject

The concept of *zero reject* provides for the education of all handicapped children. No handicapped child may be excluded from an education because of a handicap. The principle of zero reject covers both types of exclusion previously used with handicapped children; literal and functional exclusion. *Literal exclusion*—the procedure whereby handicapped children were prohibited from attending public school classes because of a handicap—is prohibited, since the law requires that all children with each state's compulsory age range be provided an education. Since the rights to an education also include that the education be "appropriate," *functional exclusion* (placing handicapped children in a program that is designed so that few or no educational benefits are received) is prohibited.

The policy of zero reject also includes a child-find program. This is divided into three components: (1) an awareness campaign, (2) location and identification of all handicapped children, and (3) diagnosis, evaluation, planning, and placement of each handicapped child into a free appropriate public education program.

Nondiscriminatory Evaluation

Assessment (testing) is essential in the schools if they are to identify, plan, and develop programs and evaluate handicapped students. A problem has been the misuse of evaluation instruments and procedures, resulting in misclassification and misplacement of handicapped students.

In P.L. 94-142, Congress delineated "nondiscriminatory procedures" to help alleviate this problem. These procedures include:

1. Tests and evaluation materials must be in the child's native language or mode of communication.
2. The materials must be administered by trained personnel in accordance with the assessment instrument guidelines.
3. The evaluation materials must be validated for the purpose for which they are used.
4. No single procedure or instrument can be used as the sole criterion for determining an appropriate educational placement or program.
5. The evaluation must include assessments of all areas related to the suspected disability.
6. The evaluation must be made by a multidisciplinary team.

Individualized Education Program (IEP)

P.L. 94-142 requires that each handicapped child's education be appropriate to his needs. This is accomplished through a process known as the Individualized Education Program (I.E.P.).

The I.E.P. is both a process and a written blueprint of the child's educational program. This document should include:

1. A statement of the child's present level of functioning.
2. A statement of annual goals and short-term instructional objectives.
3. A statement of the specific educational and related services to be provided the child and the extent of the child's participation.
4. The projected initiation dates for the services and their anticipated duration.
5. Appropriate evaluation procedures, criteria, and time lines.

Least Restrictive Environment

According to this section, handicapped children are to be integrated and educated with nonhandicapped children to the greatest degree possible. These children also cannot be removed from a regular classroom unless their handicap is such that an appropriate education cannot be achieved. A continuum of alternative placements and services must be available. When considering an alternative placement, the proximity to the students home must be considered.

Procedural Due Process

Procedural due process is the process whereby discriminatory policies may be challenged. Thus, no handicapped child can be deprived of an education without the process or mechanism to protest.

The required elements of due process included in P.L. 94-142 are as follows:

1. Written notification must be provided to the family before an evaluation. This includes the right to an interpreter or translator if the family's native language is not English—unless it is clearly not feasible.
2. The provision of written notification to the family or guardian when initiating or refusing to initiate a change in educational placement.
3. The opportunity to present complaints regarding the identification, evaluation, placement, or provision of a free, appropriate education.

4. The opportunity to obtain an independent evaluation of the child.
5. Access to all relevant records.
6. Opportunity for an impartial due process hearing which includes the right to receive timely and specific notice of any hearings; the right to be accompanied by council or professionals; the right to confront, cross examine, and call witnesses; the right to present evidence, including written or electronic records of the hearing and/or written findings of fact.
7. The right to appeal any decision and/or findings of the hearing.

Parent Participation

Parent participation is sometimes *referred to as shared decision making.* Prior to P.L. 94-142, school officials were free to make placement and programmatic decisions about handicapped children without any parental involvement. Through the I.E.P. process and due process procedures, parental involvement provisions are incorporated into P.L. 94-142. Although parents are not forced to become involved in their child's education, this section furthers the rights of those parents who do wish to involve themselves in the educational program of their child.

10

Leaving School: Educational and Work Opportunities

LEAVING SCHOOL

Handicapped children, like all children, can leave school when they are sixteen years of age. But although some disabled children wish and are ready to leave school at sixteen, many others will remain behind their fellow students. They will have missed long periods of formal education through hospital admissions, illness, and attendance at special clinics for treatment of various kinds. They may be socially immature, because they lacked the opportunities to extend their own experience and meet a variety of people. The local schools still have a duty to provide education up to the age of twenty-one if parents or children require it, but unfortunately there is frequently a shortage of places in special schools and the disabled child will often therefore have to leave.

Some handicapped children will, of course, leave school at sixteen because their parents feel unable to continue to support them in an educational setting.

A study of 788 handicapped school leavers, carried out in 1972 (*Handicapped School-Leavers: Their Further Education, Training and Employment.* Tuckey, Linda, et al., National Foundation for Educational Research, Slough, U. K.), found that only 8 (1 percent) went on to some form of higher education. None of these 788 school leavers was severely mentally handicapped. Of those who *did* get further education, the majority were blind. Only 3 out of 247 (1 percent) of the physically handicapped enjoyed this facility. Clearly facilities for academic education were better in schools for the blind. For the physically handicapped, it is likely that the practical problems of transport and access to buildings and special facilities like modified toilets, and so forth were strong deterrents.

Career counselors offer the first link between the outside world and school. All local education authorities provide vocational guidance for people in full- or part-time education. The career counselor should help in planning school career program and should meet handicapped students in or before their last year at school. Many schools also have career teachers, who can coordinate with career officers in making some realistic proposals for the handicapped school leaver.

Career teachers and counselors, in conjunction with the handicapped student, his family, and the school as a whole, will have to decide between immediate vocational training, employment, or further education. Some students are recommended to attend industrial rehabilitation units and assessment courses, or specialized residential courses. Others go on to study at a university or a college of further education (full-time or part-time), evening school, or through home tuition and correspondence courses; others attend training centers run by the local authority, which offer diversionary employment or social training only. Many school leavers will spend time in more than one of these categories, but it is clearly sensible to try to avoid wasting time on unsuitable options.

In some schools, career education and guidance may offer actual work experience for the fourteen- to sixteen-year-old age group. This work experience may take place in industrial units inside the school or in outside programs observing factory and office practices. Work orientation is particularly important for handicapped students, because they may have little experience with the normal working world and may, in addition, have problems in coping with the normal eight-hour working day.

Since one of the purposes of integration is to let the handicapped individual remain unlabeled, the counselors may not be brought in to advise on the problems of a particular disability. In this case, parents—while appreciating the normality and anonymity of the school—should ask to see a counselor. Career guidance for the disabled is a special affair, and it is essential to know the various options that are open.

ASSESSMENT FOR THE FUTURE

Some handicapped school leavers are not ready to make the transition from school to higher education or work without some intermediary process. They may have been socially restricted by frequent hospitalization. The transition from the ordered and caring atmosphere of the special school to the profit-motivated and competitive outside world may be a bewildering and frightening experience. If they have had limited curriculum and other educational opportunities, they will be greatly disadvantaged in making any realistic choices about the future. And some very severely handicapped students may have to spend so much time acquiring basic self-care skills that they are not able to apportion sufficient time to academic studies.

Traditional rehabilitation and assessment centers need to function in a different way, evaluating physical function at a particular point in time for lack of extended observation facilities, and some adolescents will, of course, attend medical rehabilitation centers, where the special facilities are essential for handicaps such as paraplegia or postaccident conditions. When a school leaver is multiply handicapped, there are very special problems in making assessments and considered judgments about future plans.

Specialist Skills for the Severely Handicapped

Many severely handicapped school leavers are simply not able to achieve higher education without an opportunity to acquire educational qualifications in a special educational setting. Because the most severely handicapped adolescents still have major communication and access problems, they may have to attend very specialized units.

Parents should therefore explore all possibilities to ensure that their child has achieved the maximum success from his school environment and that he has the opportunity to develop in the

189

future. There are a number of special colleges which meet the social, vocational, and assessment needs of handicapped school leavers.

THE DISABLED SCHOOL LEAVER
IN HIGHER EDUCATION

Although the number of disabled students has increased—corresponding to a general increase in educational opportunities for school leavers and mature students in general—there is little room for complacency. A British survey found that only 34 percent of disabled school leavers considered by their teachers to be capable of benefiting from further education actually achieved it. There is, in fact, a complex series of variables which will dictate not only acceptance at a university or college, but career achievement in the post-secondary careers.

School leavers wishing to continue their education usually have three basic options. They can attend vocational or technical schools, colleges of education (for teacher training), or universities.

Some disabled students wishing to teach will, of course, fall within the category of university entrants rather than applicants to colleges of education. Some universities regularly accept disabled applicants. These universities or colleges have extensive modifications to provide access, and normally offer special facilities such as adapted halls of residence. But some students feel strongly that they do not wish to be segregated in special accommodations within an institute for further education, and that the opportunity for social contact is quite as important as the formal academic education offered.

Making an Application

Most special schools and other schools in the community make strenuous efforts to get a disabled student accepted for higher education. Some will argue—in order to ensure that the application is considered on its individual merit—that no mention of disability should be made at application stage and the decision should rest entirely on intellectual ability. This reasoning is understandable. It is, however, dangerous, since facilities will vary enormously within individual colleges and universities. While a disability may be seen as a private matter between the candidate and the medical department, housing staff and academic staff also need to know what special facilities are to be required. Many universities, of course, will reinforce the

190

information supplied on an application form with an interview, but many applications are accepted without personal contact, and a disabled student may find himself indisputably accepted on merit, but coping with a course in a singularly unsuitable environment. Refusing to recognize disability may in such a case actually ensure a very real inequality. Consideration of applications on individual merit is in principle praiseworthy: in practice, it is difficult to see how applications can be considered without a code of practice and the establishment of guaranteed minimum standards of access to university facilities.

Very few disabled students (except perhaps for those with the most severe handicaps who will need a high degree of support in everyday living) will wish to spend their undergraduate days in a segregated situation. But it may be preferable to live with a group of disabled students in a specially built dormitory if the alternative is unsuitable and inaccessible accommodation in a university which has made few concessions to the handicapped. The choice will in the end be a personal one. Students are almost always friendly, constructive, and helpful—but the disabled student may have to accept in certain circumstances that his own privacy and independence will be lost if he has to rely too heavily on fellow students to help him move around the campus.

Getting Used to the University

Going to a university may be a major success, but a rather frightening experience nevertheless for many disabled students. Those coming from special schools will live in a fully integrated setting for the first time. Parents would do well to remember that higher education has its social as well as its academic side, and the student who has had a wide range of social experiences and is as self-sufficient as is compatible with his handicap, will find the transition from home much easier. Parents may also inadvertently place a good deal of pressure on a handicapped student to do well. Doing well is important to everyone—but many disabled people feel a disproportionate obligation to compensate for their disability with intellectual achievement. Higher education should, in the long run, be directed toward vocational ends. But many students are unsure of their future career prospects, and the disabled student should also feel free to develop options. In fact many disabled students will have had severely limited opportunities to make realistic choices regarding careers *before* they arrive at the university, because of their protected upbringing.

THE DISABLED SCHOOL LEAVER:
THE TRANSITION FROM SCHOOL TO WORK

Any child, whether handicapped or not, will acquire his own perspective on a proper role in society through the family. As he develops, he will discover and develop attitudes and interests which may suggest a pattern of employment in the future. Adults will impress upon him the necessity and value of work. Both school and parents will emphasize the essential morality of work. Unfortunately, the child who has attended a special school and whose physical abilities are very limited, may not find it easy to rationalize concerning his choice of occupation. Wheelchair living may mean that he has not had the benefit of work experience courses or of the "real" world of industry and commerce. Because of physical therapy or the limitations of his disability, he may not have attended school for more than four or five hours a day. Yet in open employment eight hours are the working norm. He may never have encountered nonhandicapped people who did not make allowances for him and have special caring relationships. He may, therefore, have quite unrealistic assessments of his own capabilities and of the satisfaction to be gained in certain kinds of employment. The initial search for suitable employment may, in fact, confront him for the first time with the real limitations of his disability and with the prejudices and misunderstandings which it can arouse.

Sheltered Employment

If outside employment seems quite impossible, the small minority of handicapped school leavers who are severely or multiply disabled will have to seek alternative means of work. Because of their historical development in rural areas, many voluntary sheltered workshops are isolated, and residential accommodation is also provided. However, an increasing number of severely disabled young people are now using the sheltered workshop as a means of developing their own self-help and vocational skills, and moving back into their communities once a suitably adapted apartment is available.

All forms of sheltered employment raise certain key questions. While sheltered employment can and should be recognized as offering opportunities to many to practice work skills and gain experience relevant to open employment, there is a temptation for workshop managers to retain their most able workers. It is difficult to offer any kind of career structure within a sheltered workshop because most supervisory and management posts will be held by able-bodied people. This is an area which could be expanded to include disabled people with management skills.

At present it seems probable that far more people would like to attend sheltered workshops, however low the pay and limited the range of occupations, than can currently be accommodated. Most disabled people, however severely incapacitated, wish to work. Work is seen not only as providing an economic reward but as conferring status upon the individual concerned.

LIVING AWAY FROM HOME

Few parents of able-bodied children think very carefully about the time when their children will leave home. They regard this as a natural occurrence which will happen in due course and are unlikely to feel that they will have any decisive power in settling the child's future life style. Disabled children, of course, present quite a different picture. The parents are likely to feel intense anxiety about their ability to cope alone: They will be frightened of the consequences of any minor accident, a fall, burning pans, and domestic disasters which might be difficult to cope with single-handed. On the other hand, they are quite naturally aware that their disabled child will probably outlive them, and they know that some provision must be made.

Many children simply continue to live at home. If the house or apartment has been suitably modified, this is the simplest solution. Perhaps it is possible to create a self-contained living unit within the home which will combine the best of all possible worlds. Otherwise, particularly if the child needs considerable assistance in day-to-day living, the parents will continue to function exactly as they did when the adult man or woman was a small child. Plainly parents who get older and frailer must be rational about their own ability to continue coping. Sometimes the additional help of hoists, electric wheelchairs, moving of toilet and bathroom facilities, and the installation of a lift will revolutionize a house's accessibility for a disabled person. Unfortunately, many of the more severely disabled will still continue to need very specific assistance in lifting and handling and—unless the family is affluent enough to be able to buy regular help—this may not be available in sufficient quantity from a local authority.

Mobility and Wheelchair Housing

If young people wish to live away from home (and particularly if they are reasonably self-sufficient), they may manage very well in an ordinary apartment which has suitable wheelchair access and where relatively minor adaptations have been made to the kitchen and bathroom. An increasing number of young handicapped people share with able-bodied people, and this is obviously a satisfying and natural way to live. Two types of housing have been distinguished: mobility and wheelchair. The former was regarded as normal housing incorporating certain basic features such as level entrance; door widths and corridors wide enough for wheelchair access; and a bathroom and at least one bedroom at the same level as the entrance. Fundamental to this concept is the principle that there should be no extra space and cost beyond the normal standards. This type of housing is, of course, suitable only for the more active wheelchair users. For the more dependent, the concept of *wheelchair housing* was devised. This housing would offer access to all principal rooms by wheelchair and would be particularly suitable for the multiply handicapped and those with deteriorating conditions.

The severely disabled have, of course, major difficulties in establishing an independent life style. There is a lack of good sheltered housing, and the alternative is likely to be some form of institutional care. Historically there has always been a tendency to segregate disabled people from the rest of the community. This is usually (quite naturally) resented by the disabled, and public and professional attitudes are beginning to change. Unfortunately, many physically and mentally handicapped people still have to use large, often remote, hospitals or homes because there is currently no substitute, and therefore the "colony" is perpetuated in rural but very isolated surroundings. Clearly some disabled young people will need a great deal of physical care. This may be quite outside the capacity of the family, but in many cases it will not be the kind of nursing care which justifies admission to a hospital unit. All of us have intermittent medical needs, but these are usually met in the community.

Staying in the Community

Some disabled people will not be able to survive on their own, however excellent their modified housing, unless they receive practical help. This help is often most needed as a result of incontinence. Incontinence is, in fact, a major reason for admission to geriatric or other wards, because the family or the disabled person is exhausted by the problem. This exhaustion may, in many cases, be due to the fact that there is insufficient support from local services or because the family feels that they cannot ask anyone else to share the embarrassing burden.

The "embarrassing" burden is, in fact, often much worse to the affected family than it is to outsiders. An advantage of the permissive society is that natural functions are both less frightening and less abnormal than they were twenty years ago. A British plan has proven that it is perfectly possible to recruit ordinary people without nursing experience to work from four to forty hours a week (often early or late) to support disabled persons in their homes.

The idea of a "bank" of volunteers or unskilled paid workers is not a new one. The *Fokus* scheme in Sweden offers specially adapted apartments in normal housing complexes. These apartments are serviced by paid staff, who operate on the relative-substitute idea and can provide basic services. In France, the *Aides Soignantes* combine nursing and domestic services through relatively untrained employees; it is felt that the system is cost-effective in freeing more skilled staff for professional deployment and in ensuring that community help is provided. Such schemes clearly require tactful planning and handling, since professionals may feel their own expertise threatened. Initially some recipients of services may also feel embarrassed or frightened at the idea of services being provided by untrained staff. But the plans have all been successful and have undoubtedly not only met real service deficiencies but have also acted as powerful public relations exercises for the disabled themselves. Family support plans need careful planning and direction, but their overall cost is modest in comparison with the provision of similar services through other channels.

Home Health Aide Agencies

In the United States, home health aide agencies are available to assist families of physically handicapped individuals or handicapped individuals with a variety of services. Assistance with physical care, such as bathing, is provided, as well as laundry services, housecleaning, or shopping.

To access the nearest home health aide agency, the individual or parent should contact the county Vocational Rehabilitation Services director, their local physician, the county Public Health Department, the county Social Service Department, or their local hospital. These agencies usually have a list of home health aide services available in the area.

Home health aide agencies are privately funded. But they do accept Medicaid, Medicare, and private insurance reimbursement in payment for their services.

Alternatives to Hospital Accommodation

If there are no local family support plans and if a high degree of care is required, there may be no alternative but to look for residential units. Many voluntary organizations provide accommodations of a very high standard for the severely disabled. Most of the major handicap organizations have lists of residential units and can advise on their suitability.

Although most people would in principle not favor the idea of segregating individuals with handicaps, there are certain practical advantages in doing so, if a handicap requires very sophisticated electronic communications equipment or other special aids.

Some residential units also offer "sheltered workshop" employment as well as residential care. Good sheltered workshops, while no substitute for independent living in the community, nevertheless offer excellent opportunities for social and some vocational development. Many young people have never acquired the skills of managing bathing, toileting, and so forth independently until they lived in an environment where the full range of equipment is available.

Housing Associations and Sheltered Housing

Housing associations have traditionally been used mainly for housing the elderly or for certain special groups, such as unmarried mothers. Their value is that they can offer special housing to meet the needs of individuals who would not normally obtain housing through a local authority. A number of voluntary organizations have provided private accommodations for the disabled.

Housing associations need not necessarily be expensive to set up, if grants are available for modification, and many local authorities are now considering the creation of a number of special living units. The creation of more mobility and wheelchair housing is essential if the disabled are to have a realistic opportunity for independence and perhaps marriage—and if their families are to continue coping when the small child becomes an adult.

Money and the Mentally Handicapped

The provision for trust funds and bequests to ensure financial support for a mentally handicapped person is even more complex than that for ensuring the financial independence of a physically disabled individual. The mentally or physically handicapped child is the most severly handicapped of all and is likely to enter residential care when his family is unable to care for him adequately at home, or when the parents die. Advice on bequests to the mentally handicapped is not a matter for the family lawyer, unless he is particularly interested in this area of work. Trusts and wills should be drawn up in consultation with the National Association for Retarded Citizens (who have advisory papers on trusts and mental handicaps) or through a special lawyer. Banks can usually recommend specialists in the creation of *discretionary trusts*, since in the eyes of the law a mentally handicapped adult is in the same position as a normal child *below the age of majority* (that is, eighteen). What must be avoided is the temptation simply to leave a lump sum or property to a mentally handicapped person without proper consideration of the issue of executors and trustees.

When a mental handicap is involved, and when there are other children alive in the family, it should be noted that a person who lacks the mental capacity to understand the legal significance and purpose of a will *cannot make a valid will in law*. For this reason, any trust set up on behalf of a mentally handicapped person should include reference to the dispersal of any capital remaining on that person's death, to ensure that he is not regarded as dying intestate, with a corresponding loss of capital to his brothers and sisters. Thinking about wills and trusts is a gloomy affair. But it is preferable to think in time and avoid family unpleasantness in the future.

11

Personal Problems

HAVING A HANDICAPPED CHILD

The pronouncement that a much-desired baby is handicapped seems like a death knell to his parents. Although handicap is a natural disaster in most cases, it is totally unexpected. We can and do plan for certain anticipated crisis areas such as old age, illness, or unemployment. But handicap, in an era of technological obstetrics and glossy commercials promoting the perfect family, is a disaster of unimaginable magnitude. Many parents are horrified and alarmed at their own reaction to having a handicapped child. The birth even of a normal healthy baby is a stressfull as well as an exciting occasion. Thoughts of new responsibilities and new limitations and anxieties perhaps about any lack of stability in the marriage will pass through many parents' heads. No one willingly admits to these feelings of stress. We all celebrate birth. But, nevertheless, all births change the family life. The birth of a handicapped child may seem to distort it. Parents often feel guilty because their first thoughts are for themselves. Perhaps they hoped their child would be clever as they never were; perhaps they wanted an athlete, a musician, an actor—they certainly expected to have the hope of somebody rather special. Handicapped people are special too—but since most people are unfamiliar with the normality and niceness of the disabled, they feel inadequate. The parents of a mentally handicapped child may be convinced that their child will never speak, have continual temper tantrums, and destroy their home. The parents of a physical handicapped child may suppose that their child will never speak, play, or go to school. Having these thoughts—and perhaps wishing that the child would die—is perfectly natural. It is a disaster reaction and won't last. But in a big maternity ward where all the other babies seem normal and where the handicapped child's arrival is greeted with an alarmed hush, it is difficult to think of the future.

Most hospitals are now very concerned at how to tell the parents and how to help them. Everybody wants to be kind and supportive. But nothing can really compensate for time and for opportunities to talk to other parents, professionals, and voluntary organizations and to acquire information about what is in store. Unfortunately many professionals also feel pain at the birth of a handicapped child; they want to be kind and sympathetic, but they also need help. This is particularly difficult if the parents appear to reject any overtures. The parent who complains about everything, who threatens to use everybody from the anesthetist to the hospital management, and who rejects every attempt to offer help and advice will possibly be marked down as neurotic and difficult. Yet this kind of behavior is natural and normal in the early states. Most parents of handicapped children admit that in the beginning they were in a state of shock.

If a doctor has had to convince the parents that their child really is handicapped, the parents may in turn conceal their own doubts about their ability to cope with a lifelong disability by turning on the doctor. If the doctor is prepared for hostility, for rudeness, and for apparent stupidity (the parents failing to remember from one consultation to the next what was proposed for their child), he or she will find it easier to be sympathetic, and to work through the parents' feelings. The sensitive doctor—or social worker or other professional worker—will make the parents feel involved in *doing something* for the child. Parents can make magnificent therapists—if they feel that they can play a proper role. Telling a mother to take her handicapped child home and love him is useless. She may take him home and love him, but will continue to be depressed and resentful. If, on the other hand, a support unit can accompany the diagnosis with an immediate plan for action and a genuine promise that help is there for the taking, the parents can feel it is really worth making an effort. As more family support units and child development centers are provided, team support for families will increase. Although handicap is primarily a family affair, many families still feel that it must be the total concern of the medical professions. They lack confidence in their own ability to help their child, and they may in consequence appear nuisances to their general practitioner and hospital doctor with continual demands for advice and help. This behavior is also natural, although time consuming, and should be recognized for what it is—a call for a vote of confidence in the *parents'* capacity to help, and a recognition of their terrible anxiety to help the child. Sometimes parents' anxiety takes another form, and they appear overprotective and anxious with any other children. However rationally they may understand the likely cause of the disability and may know that their other children are perfectly fit and healthy, some parents will persist in their fear that something will go wrong with their children. These fears may show in excessive visits to the doctor or even in overdisciplining the other children and restricting their freedom. Again, the feeling of insecurity will usually pass, but not without difficulty. In this early period after birth and diagnosis, parents often have a desperate need for advice and support.

A major problem for any caring professional is the fact that most families have the two quite separate needs. On the one hand, they need help with the machinery of day-to-day living. They need advice on aids and appliances, help with feeding a difficult child, advice on sleeping or mobility difficulties; they may need a good deal of actual practical demonstration of how to handle a child who seems potentially fragile and easily damaged. On the other hand, they also need counselling and sympathetic and uncritical support. The latter is time consuming and may take much professional time. Parents often get things badly out of perspective; they are besieged by advice from all sides (family as well as professionals). Much of this advice will come from the land of folklore and prejudice. But it will inevitably include extreme suggestions relating to blame for an apparent genetic disaster or to institutional care. If the parents feel incompetent (particularly if it is their first child and they have no experience of the normal crises and problems of babyhood), they will probably resist advice or comment. They will need sympathy and support of a positive kind over a period of time. Most parents will feel very guilty in the face of professionals because their first thoughts are for themselves.

They may have a very real need to mourn the "death" of the normal child they might have had and to come to terms with the reality. This period of grieving is now accepted as a healthy rather than histrionic part of breavement, and it is almost always so with parents of a handicapped child. Unfortunately the social workers who are particularly well equipped to cope with the counselling needs of families at crisis periods like this, often either do not know of the problem or are seen by the families as having skills only relevant to "problem families" and supplementary benefits. If the parents see particular professional skills as being relevant to members of the community whom they regard as natural losers, it may take a lot of convincing to enable them to accept their own needs for help and to understand what a social worker can offer.

All professionals are familiar with the family who firmly resists help. These "natural victims" may contact every statutory and voluntary service in an area. If they are articulate, they may well appear in the local press or on television or radio criticizing the failure of society to meet their child's needs. The battle mentality in these cases will not secure victories because the families will not accept any services which are offered. The letters to the area health authorities, the director of social services, and the local press are more a plea for help than an articulate statement of what the needs are. Some of these parents will in fact move on and become the "professional" parents who can run local groups, raise funds, and campaign for improved local facilities. This strategy of coping through helping others works well for some families.

Others will not find it so easy to take on a role within a group or to campaign publicly. Their needs may be unmet because they are unvoiced, unless there is a local system for family support. A Georgia plan (Parents to Parent), whereby the parent of a handicapped child visits each family in the maternity ward who requests it following the birth of a handicapped child and immediately offers counselling and practical advice from birth is a good one. Unfortunately, few parents get such early support, although it is almost universally true that this would have been welcomed. Because a handicap is a long-term problem, it can affect the overall development and stability of the family. As Tolstoy said in *Anna Karenina*,

"All families are unhappy in their own way," and handicapped families are also individual in their needs and disappointments. It is, however, very important that parents have the courage to ask for help when they need it and to try to be frank with the professional concerned. Sometimes it helps to write feelings or ideas down on a piece of paper, since the traditional interview is not conducive to frank discussion. Some families may find other parents helpful and supportive—although some parents feel that they cannot freely admit negative feelings to other parents in case they are "judged" by them. Parents' groups, where feelings are mutually discussed, can be immensely supportive but need skilled leaders. These are available in some areas and have the advantage of usually involving fathers *and* mothers.

THE FAMILY UNIT

When a handicapped child is born, the family will have to revise its relationship with the wider family and the community. Many parents with handicapped children tend to isolate themselves at home. This will be partly due to the sheer problem of mobility, if there is no car available. It may also be because many handicapped children have periods of physical illness and of convalescence after orthopedic or other surgery, or may be considered socially unacceptable because of behavior problems or uncontrolled epileptic seizures. In some cases, this cutting off may be due to imaginary rather than real factors. Sheila Hewett, in her study *Handicapped Children and Their Families* (University of Nottingham Press, 1970) found that

> It seemed that feelings of isolation were much more a function of the mother's personality than of the presence of a handicapped child. . . . The plight of mothers who are lonely and who do feel cut off is very real.

Some parents go through a very natural period in which they wish to withdraw and rethink their family situation and—in many cases—their life's plans. However, it is worth remembering how easy it is to become isolated. The parents may not receive complete support from their respective families (who may choose to blame the daughter or son-in-law for something that "has never happened in *our* family"). They may feel awkward and embarrassed about displaying a child who is less than perfect, or they may be even more concerned about the embarrassment of their friends who frequently have no idea how to react.

Many parents have only to experience one unfortunate casual remark—one mother heard a local worker refer to the children on her son's school bus as the product of incest; another mother found that her neighbors on a new block thought that her athetoid spastic boy had something catching—to opt out of possibly embarrassing encounters. One mother informed casual enquirers that her spina bifida boy sitting in his pushchair was nearly two. He stayed "nearly two" until he was nearly six, despite the obvious incongruity of the situation, because she preferred to avoid explanations about why he was not walking. The few parents who had the confidence to look neighbors in the eye and talk directly about their child probably got nothing but support and interest. But the anxiety about other people's opinions—particularly in certain situations like the family medical clinic where a mother may be acutely embarrassed about undressing a child with large surgical scars or with obvious abnormalities in front of a group of inquisitive mothers with normal children—are understandable.

The Carnegie Trust, in its report *Handicapped Children and Their Families* (Dunfermline, 1964) stated that "there is a different kind of balance in the family containing a handicapped child, a restructuring of attitudes which has implications for all members of the family." This reassurance may have to take account not only of what the neighbors think—and what they should be told—but of how the family will organize its life. The age of childbearing has got progressively younger, and many families will find themselves with a disabled child when the parents themselves are still unresolved about the future. If the parents are students, or if the father is unemployed, the implications will be considerable. Many jobs are highly mobile, but mobility is difficult with a handicapped child. Services vary greatly in different parts of the country. If the child has a minority condition like spina bifida or Stills disease, he may be able to have treatment only at half a dozen centers throughout the country—so moves may mean regular journeys of over a hundred miles. The family will therefore have to decide whether the father relinquishes his job, whether the family sighs and takes to the road again—or whether the parents live separately in order that the child can live a more normal life in one place. These difficulties are not insoluble, but they indicate the need for the parents to be able to communicate directly with each other. They also emphasize the need for the father to have a proper role in the care of the child, so that any job sacrifices can be seen in the perspective of family needs rather than solely of the father's disappointment.

FATHER FIGURES

Families need fathers just as they need mothers. However, in spite of women's lib, the majority of fathers are still the family's major breadwinner and are out of the home for eight to ten hours a day during the peak periods of child care. Most mothers with young children, often living many miles from their own parents, feel periods of isolation and loneliness. But the mother of a "normal" baby has opportunities to make friends through clinic visits, playgrounds in the local park, and other neighbors with young families. These opportunities exist for the mothers of handicapped babies also. But many mothers are reluctant to take out a handicapped child and have to constantly explain why the child is different. They may feel embarrassed undressing their baby at the clinic, and they may secretly feel pain and depression at the sight of active normal children compared with their own. These secret hurts are very real, but they can be dangerous.

If the mother is choosing to spend time at home in preference to going out, she may come to believe that she alone is indispensable to her child. Overprotection is the opposite of rejection, and many mothers overprotect their handicapped children. Families are held together by and large because they satisfy the individual needs of their members. Every family is different and has different needs. But the father's role may dramatically change if the mother becomes totally immersed in her child. This self-immersion may amount to deliberate self-sacrifice, but it may virtually rewrite the marriage contract for the husband. This is particularly true if the parents have differing views of the child's handicaps and needs. We all label our children to some extent. The parents with a handicapped child also labels according to need. The mentally handicapped child may be described as "a bit backward." The physically handicapped child may be described as having "slight brain damage" instead of cerebral palsy or spina bifida. Labels can be damaging in other ways, since they may belie the degree of handicap. The mother or father who cannot accept their child's disability may invest enormous and often unproductive effort in special treatments like the Doman Delacato method. Since they are hoping for miracles, they are likely to be disappointed and perhaps quick to blame themselves for failure. In other families, the parents may disagree violently about the method of caring to be adopted. If one parent seeks residential care and the other desires home care, the stresses will be enormous on the whole family.

The father has a special role in these debates. Handicapped children, even more than normal children, need their parents. The absent or desired parent is a very real disaster. If the mother becomes totally engrossed in her handicapped child and excludes the father from helping, the marriage is bound to suffer. Equally, fathers have to accept that caring for a young handicapped child can be enormously demanding and frustrating. Mothers need encouragement to lead a normal social life, to go out, and to make contact with the wider world. If they do not, the family becomes distorted and increasingly isolated. Another reason for isolation on the father's part may be that he is not actively involved in decision making concerning the child. Hospital clinics tend to take place in the middle of the working day. Some firms are sympathetic and will permit their staff to take time off to go with the mother—which may be essential, if the child is heavily handicapped and the distance is great. But if the father cannot attend clinics and physical therapy sessions or visit special schools, he will inevitably be excluded from his child's pattern of care. Both parents therefore need to make special efforts to ensure that they discuss what is decided at assessments and hospital visits, and that they are both fully aware of their child's needs and development and can act together.

BROTHERS AND SISTERS

Brothers and sisters are often supportive and concerned in the care of their handicapped sibling. But they have their own problems in "living with handicap" and in accepting that one member of the family will always have to receive what may be felt to be an unjustly large slice of the cake. Parents are often quite unaware of the conflicting feelings and emotions of their other children. Children are not normally hostile to physical disability; in fact, they have an enormous capacity for unprejudiced feeling toward anybody they like (or dislike). However, young children may be very jealous of any physical disability which seems to bring their handicapped sibling special favors and ensures that they get inadequate attention and affection. Jealousy may show itself in showing off or in aggressive or disruptive behavior (breaking toys, squabbling, shouting) in order to attract attention. Unfortunately, disruptive and attention-seeking behavior is difficult to cure once begun, and the other children's needs must be clearly observed and recognized from the beginning. Psychosomatic pains, tantrums, stealing, and clinging are all unpleasant and desperately inconvenient—particularly where the mother has a severely handicapped child to care for. The only "cure" is a more adequate rationing of time for the other children. One family created a large timetable in the kitchen on which they marked "Timothy's evening," "Jane's evening," and so forth, and ensured that the older children *did* have an evening of full attention and involvement. The creation of time for individual attention can be an enormous difficulty. It may necessitate asking neighbors to baby-sit, arranging for the handicapped child to attend a special club, or actually paying for additional assistance in the house. In some cases, it may mean letting the handicapped child have more independence and do more things with the rest of the family. Many wheelchair children are babied long after they are capable of a good degree of self-care, and it is important that they learn to be equal with their brothers and sisters.

A frequent bone of contention is the sharing of household chores. There is no reason why most handicapped children should not do their share. Admittedly there may be water spilled, and dusting will be limited to the reach of a wheelchair arm, but there are wide ranges of household gadgets available in stores which are suitable for elderly or disabled people. All children are manipulative, and the intelligent disabled child is equally capable of using his disability as a device for attracting favors and attention. This form of communication is disastrous for a handicapped child, and it is essential that the family tries hard to be scrupulously fair in its treatment of all the children.

Sometimes brothers and sisters will become very anxious and clinging, because they have failed to understand why and how the handicapped child is disabled. They may become very worried by frequent hospital visits and secretly fear that they will also become disabled and ill. Children whose brother or sister became handicapped as a result of illness and accident have, in particular, a major task in trying to come to terms with a normal child who has dramatically and suddenly become different. They may become terrified of road accidents, of doctors, or hospitals, and desperately seek reassurance. Unfortunately, this type of behavior tends to occur when the mother is already frantic with worry and inclined to think she has more than enough worries without adding to them. But failure to meet these needs for emotional reassurance may lead to truancy from school, stealing in the classroom, bullying and teasing in the street. Parents may need to examine their own feelings very carefully. Instinctively they are likely to be angry at the naughty children's lack of feeling and consideration. They are lucky to be well and able, and it seems grossly unjust that they should add to the parental burden. However, punishing children for attention-seeking behavior is unlikely to be successful. The punishment will, in its own way, be a reward, since the child will at least have attracted attention for a time. Punishment will additionally confirm the punished child's conviction that the handicapped child is the most important member of the family.

Such extremes of rivalry will not, of course, always occur. But parents need to be alert for danger signals and conscious of their other children's needs. In families where communication is good, the parents and children may be able to discuss the problem and seek some compromise solution. In some cases, the able-bodied children may actually enjoy having greater responsibility for their handicapped brother or sister. In other cases, they may wish to be relieved of the burden of pushing the wheelchair to the stores, or they may have difficulties in deciding what to say about the handicap to friends. Sometimes family conferences will help all concerned see that bad mistakes are sometimes made for the best of reasons. One family always sent the three children of the family to bed together, because the handicapped child needed plenty of rest. This "fairness" was regarded as grossly unfair by the older sisters and created enormous resentment. In another case, the fear of epileptic seizures caused the parents to forbid their other three boys to make any noise, fight, or play near their handicapped sister in case they triggered off a seizure. There was no medical basis for their fears, but it required considerable encouragement from both the pediatrician and the social worker for them to allow the other children to play normally and act as children.

Sometimes the pressure goes the other way, and the able-bodied child is inadvertently encouraged to be a "perfect" child in compensation for his brother or sister. Particularly if the handicapped child is mentally handicapped, there is often subtle pressure on the other children to do well at school, to achieve the sporting and academic progress that the parents want their children to achieve. The children themselves usually respond, but, if success is difficult to achieve, they in turn become despondent or resentful.

The usually good child who makes few demands on friends and family and who is compliant and hard working in all respects may sometimes be a very disturbed child. The brother or sister who dotes on the handicapped child, who is constantly plying the child with small attentions, may do this through love. He is also very likely to be doing it either because he is overanxious about the child (perhaps being frightened of hospital visits, death, or more imaginary disasters), or because he actually feels like being the reverse of kind. Jealousy may be carefully concealed beneath caring behavior—since many children will be acutely upset at the thought of envying a handicapped sibling. But if the jealousy is there and unrecognized, there may be problems in the future.

Clearly many families do not experience major problems in family relationships because of their handicapped child. Their relationships are good and bad at times, as in any family. But bad relationships can occur, particularly if a child needs constant and considerable attention. The parents, becoming preoccupied, may forget that communication is important and conveniently overlook other children's needs. It is always important, both for the handicapped and other children, to encourage visitors and friends to come to the house. It is easy to shut the front door; it is much harder to open it. Occasionally other children in the family may feel sensitive about having a handicapped sibling—they may have been teased at school (often innocently when somebody called them "retarded" or "spastic" with no idea of the cruelty of the taunt). If they have reached the stage of the first "date," they may wonder what to tell the new girl or boy friend. They may simply be ashamed because they are asked to do jobs around the house which they would not be asked to do if all members of the family were able-bodied. Adolescence is always a time of self-appraisal, and most teenagers occasionally look at their family through less than rose-colored glasses. Particularly if a handicap is known to be congenital (such as hemophilia), great tact may be needed in supporting an adolescent girl who suddenly wonders if she will ever be able to have babies—or an adolescent boy who is secretly worrying what the new girl friend will think of the cerebral palsied brother who cannot talk intelligibly. Fortunately, attitudes are changing and television in particular has made most people more tolerant and more understanding of people with a handicap. Parents owe it to themselves and their children to be able to be straightforward about it, its cause, and its treatment.

CHILDHOOD INDEPENDENCE

Parents can also help their child by ensuring that their home is a warm and friendly place for young people to visit. Children may stare at a wheelchair in the street. They will look quite differently if they are invited into the house and shown that disabled people are quite ordinary people with a disability. Often the parents themselves are the barriers to this kind of integration, because they are frightened of the children being hurt. But the advantage of childhood is that all questions can be asked directly, and that factual answers can be accepted without disgust. Children often do ask questions about incontinence, braces, and the causes of handicap which parents would prefer to remain unanswered. But their interest is direct and practical. and their curiosity should be satisfied.

Some parents worry enormously about wheelchair children who wish to play in the road or neighboring yards with their friends. Many disabled children are very mobile in their chairs or on adapted tricycles, and it is essential that they should be allowed to take some risks in order to make friends and develop new skills. Although there is a real risk of fractures for a few children, it is essential that the desire and determination to get out into the community should be recognized.

Older children can learn to go on simple errands to local stores and houses. They need to learn road sense like all children (and more than some, since they may have little opportunity to experience much traffic risk). It is important for children to go and buy their own magazines, call for their friends, or simply go down to the local football field *on their own* as soon as they feel able. Nervous parents might remember that, although possibly rather more fragile than other children, a disabled child is an obvious object and so is unlikely to get lost without a trace, or to be hit by an unseeing car on a street crossing. But, since wheelchairs can move at considerable speed on suitable slopes, it is also essential to impress on the child the need for care and caution both on public sidewalks and when crossing roads.

THE CHILD'S PERCEPTION OF HIS HANDICAP

Handicapped children amy take some time to accept that their disability is lasting and permanent. Because so many children with major physical handicaps have frequent orthopedic operations and hospital visits, it is tempting and natural for them to believe that eventually they will be whole and healthy. Jane was one such child who had extensive surgery for spina bifida. The result of the surgery was that she would walk slowly and for limited periods with braces and crutches. In view of the severity of her handicap, the achievement was considerable. But Jane had spent most of her early life in the hospital or a special school. As a result, she was convinced that it was only children who were handicapped: When they grew up, they would be like other able-bodied adults. When she reached early adolescence and was forced to accept that there would be no more operations and no "cure," she went through a period of profound depression before coming to terms with her disability. Jane was lucky; she had a caring and supportive family. But some families perpetuate the notion of an eventual cure because they themselves wish to believe it. A study carried out in 1961 among 128 children with cerebral palsy asked the children to make three wishes. The wishes relating to handicap and cure came only from the older children (on average fifteen years)—an indication of the number of physically handicapped children who do not become seriously aware of the permanence of their handicap until early adolescence. Denial of handicap and overexpectation about possible career options are perfectly natural and something that most children experience. But fantasies are dangerous if they are perpetuated, and parents sometimes accidentalyy encourage them by suggesting to the child going into the hospital that the forthcoming treatment will make a major improvement. The "let down" feeling when there is no obvious improvement may be considerable.

Another problem may lie in the child's overprotection from birth, which makes him feel quietly inferior and incompetent in the presence of the able-bodied. Handicapped children must learn to face challenge, particularly if they go to a normal school. They are more likely to do this if demands have been made on them at home, and they are anxious to learn new skills. Sometimes parents may have to tactfully divert interests or encourage different skills. The boy who cannot manage football because of braces and poor coordination may prove to be an excellent swimmer. If children are not allowed to participate in a range of activities (with some sort of success), they are liable to become hypochondriacs and use their handicap as an excuse not to try. Sometimes teachers with little knowledge of physical handicap increase this difficulty by constantly removing a child from the scene of action in case he falls, breaks a brace, or falls out of his wheelchair. If this is the case, the parents must tactfully try to explain what the child can do, how much freedom he can be given, and what he *wants* to do, so that he can be encouraged into joining in a variety of activities. It may be up to parents sometimes to say that *they* don't mind the child's trousers and parka being coated with mud, that they are quite happy to see scuffed shoes, and that they will not blame the school if he comes home with bumps and bruises. Physically handicapped children are bound to have stressful experiences; they will need additional determination to master their environment. But happiness is not found in avoiding all stressful activities, and parents need to balance out what their child can be asked to do—and what is too demanding and frustrating to increase his skills or enjoyment.

THINKING ABOUT DEATH

Anxiety and stress are of course quite different where a child has a degenerative illness and realizes that he will get worse and eventually die. The family's problem in deciding whether to tell the child, how to tell other relatives and friends, and how to come to terms with their own feelings, are very real. All too often professionals, doctors included, avoid any discussion of death and its aftermath. Children themselves vary in the ages at which they become truly conscious of death as the end of life, and not as a kind of magical disappearance like going to sleep or going away. The researchers of Sylvia Anthony suggests that children begin to be conscious of death at about five, but that it is not until they are about nine years old that they really acquire a rational idea of death. At this age death is more fearful— because it is related to real people—and the bereaved child will grieve and mourn a dead parent or friend with the sorrow and emotion expressed also in adult life. It is known that children with chronic handicaps or illnesses are more prone to develop psychiatric disorders than other children. The fact is not surprising, since they are living with constant tension. The child who is already disturbed will be increasingly disturbed if he is afraid of death. Often adults falsely assume that children are too young to understand, and that it is better to avoid any mention of the subject. Unfortunately, death is more taboo than sex, violence, religion, or any of the formerly sensitive areas in our society. Precisely because many people will not see death or attend a funeral until well into adult life, parents themselves may be terrified. Most deaths take place in hospitals, and the ritual

211

of the medieval "good death" is long forgotten. There is therefore no natural way to react, as families instinctively react to childbirth or marriages.

Parents may feel a great deal of guilt that their child is dying. They may blame themselves for not having recognized the genetic risk of muscular dystrophy (although usually there is no way of anticipating this congenital handicap). They may feel that their care and nursing has been inadequate, and they can feel enormously unhappy if the child's personality appears to change in the terminal stage of illness. Many children are peevish and unhappy when they are ill, and parents can feel that they are being rejected. If a child becomes gradually more handicapped, a decision may have to be made about who will care for him. Many muscular dystrophy children become severely handicapped in adolescence. If several boys in a family are affected, the physical problems of care may be astronomical. In some cases, it may be essential to share the burden.

If there are other children in the family, it can be very difficult to know whether to involve them in the situation. Very young children will not understand (except in the sense that they may develop inexplicable fears about hospitals, doctors, and people disappearing). Older children, like their parents, will have to go through what Freud called "the work of mourning." They will grieve and have to come to terms with their grief, sense of loss, and perhaps guilt. Since death and mourning are becoming increasingly solitary affairs, children may find themselves totally excluded from any discussion of their feelings. The bereaved parents will be expected to shut themselves away and mourn; the surviving children will be cared for by relatives or neighbors who will be kind but almost always reluctant to discuss what has happened. Some children will worry that they may share their dead sibling's fate. They imagine aches, pains, and physical symptoms. Other children may be overwhelmed by guilt. Perhaps they secretly disliked or were jealous of the dead child. They may bitterly have resented the increasingly limitations on family activities, the tiredness of the parents, the feelings that *they* did not matter. Rationally they will have understood why life was like it was. But irrationally they may have made remarks or expressed wishes that they now wish unsaid. Many children secretly half believe in magic and mystical powers; they may feel that they have produced a kind of "curse" on the dead child and that the death is their fault. If the origins of the handicap or illness have never been discussed, it is not surprising that they are confused. Often parents are quite incapable of dealing with these feelings because of their own grief. Sometimes a sensitive family friend or other relative can comfort a child, give him the opportunity he needs to discuss what has happened, and help him accept that he is not to blame. A child who cannot discuss these feelings may continue to feel (because of his parents' preoccupation with grief) that he is superfluous to the family and become more resentful and sad. Parents have to learn to accept their own negative feelings toward themselves and the dead before they can help their living children.

Since death is always presented as a bloody and violent affair on the television screen—and few young children now see an elderly person die quietly and with dignity at home—there may be a genuine fear about *how* death comes. Children may imagine that the doctor "does something" or that the hospital hides harrowing scenes. Children do not need medical definitions, but can be reassured that death can be a tranquil and peaceful affair despite the array of hospital machinery with which a dying person is often surrounded. Some agnostic parents worry about their children's easy acceptance that "dead people go to heaven" or become angels. Most young children find abstract attitudes hard to grasp, and heaven is a convenient way of "going somewhere." If children find this explanation of death helpful—or if their parents also have the religious convictions to share it—there is no need to enter into speculation on life after death. It is not fair to ignore the problem and hope reassurances will work, if the sick child or his brothers and sisters clearly wish to discuss it. if children develop protective ideas of heaven, angels, and everlasting life, it is unnecessary to shatter these thoughts with detailed scientific explanations.

GROWING UP—THE OTHER SEX

Adolescence is a time of turmoil for all children. Many will feel uncertain of their own personal value and experience periods of doubts about their own worth and self-image. Many able-bodied children will, indeed, feel that acne, overweight, or poor eyesight are real disabilities that render them undesirable in the eyes of their contemporaries: It is very difficult to grow up in a society where physical appearance matters so much. The media and television all express the stereotyped glossy image. Sexuality is "sold" with every commodity, and the handsome, competent, and active man and woman stares out at anyone who is less than confident of their own personal value. Handicapped children are also susceptible to the images projected by the media. Indeed, precisely because they are limited by a physical disability, they may be even more susceptible to fantasies and day dreams. Although a physically handicapped girl may be very well aware that she cannot do the latest dance step and the handicapped boy may understand that he is unlikely to leap onto a motor bike and win the next lap, they may also have a contradictory self-image of the people they would like to be. The "Billy Liar" self-projection is common among *all* adolescents. In itself, it is harmless. If it becomes fixed, it has dangers.

Sexuality is much more than sex. It is part of basic communication, and mature young men or women instinctively express a consciousness of sexuality and of their own personality in all their relationships. Unfortunately sexuality and sex have been confused in the minds of many parents and professionals. Parents of a handicapped child may actually secretly feel relief that this child "won't worry me." They feel that wheelchair living is incompatible with a normal sexual relationship. Indeed, they may feel embarrassed at the thought that a disabled person should actually wish to have a sexual relationship. This is, of course, partly due to the immense concern which parents feel for a handicapped child. Precisely because they feel that no one could feel "that way" about a handicapped boy or girl, they are sure their child will be exploited in any sexual relationship. They cannot imagine a normal able-bodied man or woman wishing to initiate a relationship, except for confused and unhealthy reasons. They may feel that a relationship between two disabled people is equally unnatural. Indeed, they may feel that this relationship (which is initially the most probable, since a physically handicapped adolescent is more likely to meet other handicapped adolescents at school or at clubs) is threatening to *them.*

Parents of normal children look forward to the end of adolescence and a relief from responsibility. Of course, no parent is ever entirely free from concern. A mother will worry about her daughter's asthma, a father about his son's fast driving when the children concerned are middle-aged. But adolescence is a watershed, and after the storms and turbulence are over, a happier, more settled relationship can be eagerly anticipated. Having a child with a handicap may cheat parents of this comfortable relationship with mature children. The parent may not be able to anticipate grandchildren. If they accept that their child *can* bear children, they may be terrified of the responsibility to *them* if a son or daughter cannot cope with an active toddler or infant.

Parents may very well feel that no one will care for their child as they have done: supply the balanced diet, attend to laundry, transport, and cope with depression. In addition, parents who have lived for a lifetime with a handicap may have sustained their own role by accepting the very special caring relationship which can develop between parents and a dependent handicapped child. This "love and care" is, of course, experienced by all parents in the toddler period. It is often a "love and hate" relationship, since the demands of care and attention have to be offset against the personal attachment and bonding with the parent. It is a close, intimate relationship which growing up and going to school will naturally change and shape into something more interdependent. But this process of growth and development may never have occurred with parents of handicapped children. If the child has a real lack of self-help skills, the parents will probably have shouldered a heavy and constant burden of care. However willingly this has been given, the parents will inevitably have sacrificed some of their own activities and relationships. Their own social life and relationships will probably have narrowed, and they may in turn depend upon the affection and intimacy which exists with the handicapped child. If this child forms another close relationship, falls in love, and considers marriage, they may feel alienated and even jealous. This is particularly understandable in view of the fact that a failed relationship will be much worse for a handicapped child than for a normal one, who can more easily rush off and seek a new partner. And a possibly scarred self-image will have received yet another blow. It should, of course, be added that residential child-care staff also have the same vulnerability to this withdrawal of love and transfer of affection. Both they and parents need to examine their own feelings frankly and honestly with regard to the adolescent.

Sex is quite possible for the vast majority of handicapped children. It is true that there may be some physical difficulties to be resolved, but even quadriplegia (paralysis of four limbs and trunk) is not a barrier. The majority of paraplegic women will be able to have children, and contraception is as relevant to them as to all other members of the community.

Where a handicapped child may have real difficulties is in his attitudes to and knowledge of sex. A child in a wheelchair is physically restricted. However well-adapted his home, there will be little opportunity for privacy with other adolescents. Attendance at clubs will involve parental transport or group trips in a minibus. The kind of informal and (to parental ears) crude exploratory talk which is quite normal in able-bodied adolescents is unlikely to occur. Farmyard jokes may irritate parents and teachers. But they have their own place in trying out ideas and facts. Physical isolation may also mean that wheelchair adolescents get little opportunity to observe the natural patterns of courtship and bonding, pairing up at dances and coffee bars, casual conversation, and group activities. Their knowledge of appropriate behavior for men and women may be based upon improbable soap box dramas on television or upon books and journals. In any event, they may develop grossly unrealistic ideas about human behavior. Because of conflicts in their own feelings and the images of "desirable" behavior as perceived at school or in the media, they may even adopt extremely moral and censorious attitudes toward anything sexual. This is often a form of self-defense. As one physically handicapped teenage boy commented, "No one went into a convent in the Middle Ages unless they *thought* themselves ugly." A handicapped adolescent may need a good deal of help to admit his own feelings and accept that he does not have to keep to a kind of moral "purdah" as self-protection.

Information on Sex

Teachers and parents have an important part to play in seeing that a handicapped child has proper information. It is quite possible for a handicapped child to have great problems in perceiving reproduction, for example, in relation to his own disabled body. All of us, when we look in the mirror, see a number of self-images. If we are happy, we see an attractive, purposeful face. If we are depressed, we may imagine our features to be pathologically ugly and unlovable. The handicapped child will also seesaw between extremes of feeling. On the one hand, he may feel embarrassed at the idea of his body. Handicapped children have, after all, seen their bodies regarded as public property over the years in hospital outpatients departments. They may have developed a clinical detachment to cope with this, which enables them to regard any dysfunction as a "mechanical breakdown" requiring objective treatment. This strategy may be more comfortable and less damaging emotionally, than allowing feelings through, but it may then become very hard for the child to switch to a more sensual and emotional approach to the human body. Sexuality is, of course, in part communication through touch and gesture. Some help may be needed to appreciate this.

There is no real substitute for talk and counselling. But if parents and teachers are inhibited, fumbled explanations and hurried talk will be of little use. There is a mass of useful printed information, which has the advantage over personal explanation that it is less likely to be misunderstood, and this can form the basis for any questions and discussion. If a child needs help, and the parents feel they cannot give it, it might be useful to seek some form of independent advocacy and counselling. Many schools now provide this as part of overall health education. If not, youth advisory services exist in many districts and can be identified through family planning clincs, doctors' offices, or mental health departments. The importance of an individual who is independent of the child's home and school environment is that he or she is much more likely to be able to present a realistic and objective picture of what will happen in the future. If a handicapped child feels embarrassed at mentioning contraception, he is much freer with a stranger and less inhibited at asking naive questions.

Contraception

If we accept the implications of sexuality in the disabled, we also have to consider practical details. Contraception advice is absolutely critical. First, anybody in a wheelchair will have much more difficulty in obtaining contraceptives or books on the subject because of problems of physical access to the appropriate stores or clinics. Second, limited social contacts will make it very improbable that a handicapped child knows much about what contraception is or what the risks of pregnancy are. Many handicapped girls are convinced that they will never get pregnant, and are woefully ignorant of the symptoms of pregnancy if it should happen. Some parents might contend that the subject was better left alone, because of embarrassment and because of the relaxation of restrictions on abortion facilities. But this attitude ignores the fact that many handicapped girls will desperately want a child of their own. Childbearing will prove their normality and identity as a woman—a healthy child will to some extent diminish their own feeling of disability and will also be seen as a source of love and attention. Needless to say, agreement to an abortion will be very difficult and filled with emotional problems in a case of this kind. The strains on the family will be enormous. Parents will feel quite unable to care for a baby as well as a dependent daughter. The daughter will be terrified that she will never have another chance to have a child. It is certainly *not* safe to assume that a girl in a wheelchair cannot get pregnant. Emphasis should be placed on personal responsibility and (if necessary) family planning advice sould be obtained. If a girl is very physically handicapped, this advice may need to be specialized. But the pill, if medically approved, has the enormous advantage for a disabled girl in regulating the menstrual cycle and thus minimizing what can be a major problem for somebody with limited physical mobility.

Many physically handicapped children complain when they reach adolescence, that they wish to see their doctors alone without parents present. Parents should try to meet this desire (which may give the only private opportunity to discuss problems of a sexual nature) and accept the dilemma of children who are almost adult but who have to accept an often humilating degree of dependence on their parents.

GETTING MARRIED

Relationships with the opposite sex need not mean marriage. In fact, it may be realistic to assume that a number of handicapped people will not be able to get married because of problems of immaturity, illness, or lack of self-care skills. In fact, a handicapped person may be totally unaware of the basic facts of day-to-day living in marriage. If a child has been away at school or if the parents have discouraged any very active participation in running the home, he may be quite unaware of the different stages of producing regular meals, of how to clean a floor, or of how to mend a shirt. He may not have thought of the difficulties of managing shopping and transport, or indeed of managing in those situations where an able-bodied arm is useful.

There are increasing numbers of apartments and houses adapted for the handicapped, and independence is a very real possibility. But even this presupposes *practical* knowledge of budgeting and home management. These skills will generally be acquired in a hit-and-miss manner by able-bodied adolescents. But *they* have the physical mobility to experiment with living in squalor, and it is much more difficult for an individual in a wheelchair to learn through mistakes, when each mistake may have taken such a long time to perform. In this sense, parents have a very real responsibility to encourage their child to participate fully in running the house. It is much easier to decide for him that such and such a meal will appear on the table on Monday and that sheets will be changed on Tuesday. But these "survival" routines for the rest of the family encourage inertia. Certainly no wheelchair adolescent should be encouraged to marry until he has genuinely and thoroughly considered his own ability to assume responsibility and the practical implications for the new family unit.

Many parents may secretly hope that their disabled child will marry a sympathetic, charming, and above all *able-bodied* partner, who will perpetuate the parental role when they can no longer sustain it. They have reason in their hopes, since a large number of disabled people do marry able-bodied partners. However, precisely because divorce is so humiliating and hurtful to a handicapped person, any consideration of marriage requires very frank discussion. If the disability is congenital, genetic counselling should be obtained to avoid the possibility of future recriminations or heartbreak. Many men and women actively enjoy providing the extra support that a handicapped partner needs. But if the handicapped person is seeking a lover and the able-bodied partner a child, the relationship can be doomed to failure. All marriages are, of course, risks. But where there is a handicap, the financial, emotional, and social implications need to be discussed very fully.

A very real problem for parents may occur when a handicapped child desperately yearns for an able-bodied partner to establish his or her own normality. A rather isolated handicapped child may have very lofty and romantic perceptions of marriage and love, and may in fact pursue a quite impossible dream. All of us dream—and we are surely entitled to romanticism in our lives. But this romanticism should not obscure the realities of life and cut an individual off from other relationships. Precisely because they are more likely to meet each other, disabled men and women are more likely to marry. Two disabilities do not necessarily compound a problem, since modified housing can provide a suitable environment, and both partners will understand the other's physical limitations. The problem in this case may be that the couple may have great difficulty in establishing a relationship because of lack of privacy. The handicapped girl who wished for an able-bodied boy friend so that he could take her out on her own in his car, was expressing a very real need. Three-wheeler cars do not encourage intimacy, and even at home very few young adults will be able to have much privacy.

It should perhaps be said, in conclusion, that the best thing parents can do for their handicapped children—apart from the obvious love and support which they give so willingly—is to encourage their overall maturity and development so that they can make their own decisions. We can all laugh at the often quoted "does he take sugar in his coffee?" syndrome. Yet as parents of handicapped children, it is dreadfully easy to decide that "he does take sugar in his coffee" and pursue a line that is domestically convenient. Disabled children can have very confused images of themselves. They have to learn to live with a degree of dependency, and they may find this easiest to cope with in terms of compliance and inertia. But, however inconvenient to parents, they need to overcome their inherent immaturity and learn to make some of the decisons which they will need to make if they are adults in the outside world. Some children will be so handicapped that they may never be able to make many decisions realistically. But others will be capable of astonishing their parents with new skills and confidence. In all relationships, both sexual ones and those in school or work situations, communication skills are crucial. The source of these will lie in the family and, hopefully, will enrich the family in turn.

12

Leisure, Play, and Vacation Activities

Play is a way of life for all children. But exploration, even of the home environment, is often difficult for many children with a physical or mental handicap. Most young children, handicapped or not, spend the major part of their day in the home, but the normal active toddler will make constant assaults on cupboards, saucepan lids, books, shoes—any object within physical grasp. This "interference" is not, of course, naughtiness. It is a natural attempt to learn. Babies and young children need to feel things to develop their tactile senses. The squashy sensation of a sponge, the tickle of a feather duster, the clatter of two saucepan lids together are as important as access to model cars and cuddly teddy bears. If a child cannot explore because he has not reached the stage of crawling or

221

shuffling or cannot use a mobility aid, he may miss out on these normal stages of learning through play. If a child appears delicate, is constantly subject to respiratory tract infections, or has a condition such as hemophilia where bumps are dangerous, it is natural for his mother to try to protect him. The stroller or chair may seem the safest place. If a child has very limited physical ability and cannot manipulate a toy in his fingers, observation from a seat or bed may again seem the only occupation open to him.

But these children who are already deprived of experiences by their handicap, are literally at risk of further handicap if they are not encouraged to explore their environment and begin to play. The good or dull child may really be a bored child, and it is up to his parents to invent stimulating experiences for him. There is a wide range of manufactured or homemade play things that can be adapted to individual needs. Some mothers may complain, when they begin really to play with their child, that he is no longer "good," and that he makes demands for their attention. But this is really progress, when he shows that he wants them to play and relate to him, and the temporary inconvenience of a demanding child is nothing compared with the long-term advantages of a child who has been adequately stimulated and involved from birth. The baby chewing and turning the cotton spool in his fingers is acquiring fine finger control which will eventually enable him to manipulate a pen and write. The child fitting saucepan lids to pans or building with blocks is acquiring a knowledge of dimension and space which will be needed when he later has to acquire mathematical concepts. While it is true that a lively, intelligent child with full physical abilities almost always seems to acquire skills by a process of osmosis with his environment, children with handicaps will need *help*. A child with any degree of mental retardation will in particular require very active help to interest and encourage his participation in the "real" world. Play is a continuous learning process that is also *fun*. Parents and professionals need to understand how important it is to a handicapped child to develop and widen his horizons and social contacts.

What Kind of Play?

Even a newborn baby can begin to play and enjoy stimulation, and the first toys might be mobiles, which can be bought or made to encourage reactions to color and light. For a child with any visual problems, mobiles can be made which jingle or tinkle in the movement of the air. A wide range of musical boxes and other toys are

222

available that can be used in conjunction with visual toys. Hand and eye coordination is late in developing in many handicapped children, so hanging suitable brightly colored and textured toys over the bed may be of particular importance to encourage them to reach out and grasp. Needless to say, the object of any game is success, so hanging toys should be placed carefully so that the child can both see and touch. The effect of mobiles can be doubled or varied by moving the bed so that the mobile is reflected in a mirror, or so that sunlight from a window produces more glitter. Since familiarity breeds contempt, mobiles should be changed so that the child is not constantly seeing the same shapes and colors. Young children react best to toys with strong primary colors, rather than pastels. They need direct impact on their senses. Even quite small babies may also react to colorful wall hangings or posters, and these can be easily varied.

But most important of all, very young children need eye-to-eye contact and play with their parents. The traditional nursery rhymes and singing games are all important in involving the child. Children with a degree of mental handicap may be difficult and unrewarding at first when playing these kinds of games. They may appear apathetic and floppy, but involvement will come with time. There is ample research evidence to show that children need affection and involvement as much as they need food and clean clothes. It is easy to starve a handicapped child of active stimulation and affection by accident, by assuming that he is actually happier just lying or sitting there while mother gets on with her chores around the house. But a handicapped child cannot afford to be stunted by lack of interest, and he is unlikely to develop new skills without a lot of encouragement. Remember that very young or very handicapped children will be far more ready to play with their mother, their food, or their own bodies than with toys.

Special Toys

Handicapped children have the same play needs as normal children, but they may need more help in selecting toys and activities which will help them develop new skills as well as provide enjoyment. *Creative play* is an essential part of development for all children. Some handicapped children do not like messy activities and are frightened of playing with sand, finger paints, papier-maché, or dough. They may need gentle encouragement to feel, touch, mold, and play. Printing with blocks cut from potatoes is often popular and gives good results with minimal hand control. Collages, using flour and water paste, are enjoyable for a child whose finger control is too poor for fine paintwork or drawing. If cutting is impossible, different scraps of paper can be loosely cut up and pushed onto a prepasted piece of paper. Many children enjoy magnetic boards, which can be simply made for use at home by sticking magnetic tape (available from shops stocking tape recorders and other audio aids) onto shapes and figures. These figures can then be stuck to any metal surface, ranging from tin trays to the refrigerator door. Many children enjoy playing with water and will play for hours with bubble pipes, sieves, and pieces of kitchen equipment in a bowl of water. There is a wide range of protective plastic clothing available; and a wet kitchen floor is a small price to pay for a happy child and an hour or so of occupation.

Children also need toys for *fantasy play*. All children enjoy acting our their everyday experiences, and children who have been in the hospital, or who are about to go, will enjoy miniature nurse and doctor dolls. These are available from a number of manufacturers, including Schaper Playmobil and Childcraft (see Appendix B for addresses) and they come complete with wheelchairs, bed pans, and operating tables. The Fisher-Price toys are widely available and offer a range of doll houses, schools, airports, and other settings, peopled and furnished by small sturdy plastic dolls and animals. These are extremely tough and easily manipulated. Playhouses are also popular. The immobile child can be sat inside of a playhouse in a triangle or other chair or placed on the floor or on a beanbag. Children in wheelchairs get very little privacy, and the seclusion of a playhouse will offer a novel experience of being in charge of a house and feeling independent. Doll houses, simple railways, and motorway sets are all popular with both sexes and encourage talk and social play with another child. If a child wishes to play with a train layout or a large number of small toys, but cannot sit, he can be lain on the floor on his stomach over a foam wedge. This will extend his reach and enable him to roll cars and trains without the risk of dropping them off a wheelchair tray or table. If children have perceptual problems, it is particularly important that they should have opportunities for fantasy play, in order that they can learn the distinction between "up" and "down" and "here" and "over there." Parents can help by asking the child to move toys in a certain direction, or by telling a story which the child will move trains and dolls to illustrate. Small realistic toys are useful means of expanding and reinforcing basic vocabulary, and they additionally encourage the child to make fine finger movements and manipulate toys in a very limited space.

Communication toys have two purposes—to encourage speech and to stimulate a child so that he wishes to speak. Talking dolls, chattering telephones, squeaking dogs and frogs, and hooting trains amuse children and will often stimulate them to respond. Many children greatly enjoy battery-operated telephones or intercoms and will sing or talk to somebody in the next room. Cassette players are also useful. Even if a child does not recognize his own voice, he will recognize his mother's, and the sound of any musical toys. Musical toys such as xylophones, trumpets, recorders, cymbals, or any simple noise-producing instrument are equally exhilarating. Although there is a school of thought which disapproves of the unmusical use of percussion instruments or recorders, most preschool children greatly enjoy making noise. They can also be encouraged to make appropriate noises, banging a cymbal or a drum in time to music or singing, which will develop their own concentration and hearing skills.

If a child is severely handicapped, or if there are problems of mental retardation, it may be difficult to find toys which really hold interest. Something simple like a jack-in-the-box or a musical box popup toy may be successful. Alternatively some children respond to difficult textures. In the last resort it is the child who must choose and who will enjoy or reject the toy.

Many parents make the basic error of assuming that a child needs no assistance in play. Children need encouragement and initiation into many games. If the beads are not threaded or the blocks made into a tower, it may simply be that the child wishes to have an audience whose approval he can receive. Many physically handicapped children, who have had long periods of enforced immobility in a cast or in the hospital, have become quiet and withdrawn as a means of coping with their restricted environment. If they are stimulated to play, they may temporarily actually seem "naughty" or "not quite their self" to their parents. An interested child is a lively child, and will not be willing to lie quietly on the floor or sit in a wheelchair without purposeful occupation. Parents, therefore, need to recognize this aspect of child development, which they may not have consciously observed in other able-bodied children in the family. The active toddler will be constantly on the move, into every room and piece of furniture, touching and asking. The immobile child will not be able to achieve this mobility. Even with a walking aid, he will have certain physical constraints in exploration or touching. Therefore he will have to turn to his mother and ask and demand. If she sees play as a continuous baby sitter while she concentrates on the household chores, one of two things can happen: either the child will again lose interest and become apathetic and disinterested, or he will become attention-seeking and unhappy. All mothers at times naturally need to feel that they can rely on their child being happy and fully occupied while they get on with other things. But they should consciously set aside certain periods of the day for *active* play, for initiating new toys and games, and for playing *socially* wih the child.

Social play is particularly important because many handicapped children will not have casual opportunities for play with other children. The immobile child is unlikely to be invited to pop in next door for an hour or so while his mother goes shopping. If children are in the house, they may have been severely cautioned not to annoy or upset the handicapped child. As a result they may be shy and anxious not to offend. Parents can start by encouraging their child to talk and to play games which involve two people. There are a number of simple games, such as picture lotto and dominoes, which can be played from an early age. Lotto can be understood by many children from three years old. If a child is physically insecure and timid, he will need additional encouragement to accept the company of his peers.

Preschool playgroups are invaluable for handicapped children, because they offer socialization in (usually) suitable premises on a neighborhood basis. But it is sensible to reduce the problems of settling in by encouraging the child in advance to sample many of the playschool activities and games. He will then find the transitional period less terrifying and will settle down more easily. It should not be difficult to find another local child already at the playschool, who can be invited to play as a preliminary. Since children are curious but practical, they will quickly accept physical abnormalities or appliances such as braces or wheelchairs. The greater problem often lies in the mother's own anxiety and ambivalence in case her child finds social contacts unrewarding and rejecting. Fortunately, small children are sufficiently unsophisticated to avoid the failings of their elders, and they do not usually have any preconceptions about handicaps. Preschool is therefore a good age to use toys and play equipment as the basis for social relationships. It should be added that—even if a handicapped child will never use it himself—large play equipment such as climbing frames or trampolines may be useful in order to persuade other children to come in. One mother, who turned her back yard into a neighborhood playground, reported that the equipment had proved an investment, because once the children had actually come into the yard, they would devise games which involved the handicapped child. This might mean turning the climbing frame into a house with a blanket as a roof, or pushing the handicapped child around the yard in trucks and cars. Clearly some children will not be able to enjoy unrestricted outdoor play, for fear of accident or injury. But many can and will enjoy it and the small spina bifida boy with his trolley or wheelchair may prove an equal participant with his able-bodied neighbors.

PRESCHOOLS

Where there is no local special group or class, physically handicapped children may be able to attend a normal play school. Play schools, like families, vary and not all groups will have the ratio of helpers or a suitable physical environment to meet the needs of severely handicapped children. But remarkably little special equipment is usually required, since the handicapped child needs the ordinary play school facilities of access to various play experiences, social contacts, and stimulation much more than he needs specially built furniture or necessarily special toys. Some handicapped children have had unpleasant hospital experiences—a spina bifida child may have spent a large part of his preschool years in a hospital bed. As a result, the process of separation and adjustment may be more protracted than with a normal child. Because of his social immaturity, the inexperienced and handicapped child may also need to start before he has acquired the usual preschool skills of toilet training and walking, so he may need his mother's presence for much longer than a normal child. Handicapped children may need more supported play (because they may lack the motivation or stimulation to take the initiative on their own). A good play school will consider the separate but simultaneous needs of parents *and* children, and can play a major role in encouraging the *mother* to relinquish the care of her child to others.

The choice of preschool provision will depend, to a considerable extent, on the availability of local resources. But, whatever is chosen, handicapped children *need* to acquire sensory and manipulative skills before they start school. They need to learn to relate sociably to other children and adults. The United Kingdom's Pre-School Playgroups Association recognizes this:

Handicapped children are children first, with the same needs as all children, and second with special needs that arise from their handicaps. The

227

special needs are extra ones, not alternative ones to those all children share. The parents have special needs too, for they may miss some of the normal rewards and reassurance of parenthood.

HANDICAPPED ADVENTURE PLAYGROUNDS

Many handicapped children are sadly neglected with regard to provision for outdoor physical play. Play is far more than a cuddly toy, and physically handicapped children in particular have frequently been denied normal experiences for natural development because of the lack of special facilities to meet their needs. In 1966, the first Adventure Playground for Handicapped Children was established in London. It was specially designed and equipped to provide enjoyment and sensory-motor training for children with a range of disabilities. The site chosen was a large private garden, well wooded and safely enclosed but large enough to offer a sense of physical freedom. The basis of the playground's philosophy was the need to provide what the *children*, rather than the handicap, needed. Handicapped children rarely experience a completely free play situation: parents and teachers naturally protect them, overemphasize physical safety, and are very conscious of the educative role of play.

Because of their limited physical experience, disabled children need a good deal of encouragement and reassurance when they first enter a handicapped children's adventure playground. They have to acquire the confidence to explore and exploit their new environment. Such playgrounds do not segregate children but rather integrate them into the normal world of play. Very few physically handicapped children, for instance, are encouraged to get out of wheelchairs in their own yards and crawl in the mud. But the Chelsea playground has protective play clothes for "dirty" activities, for bonfires and cooking; it also has dressing-up clothes, inflatable cushions and mattresses, and trampolines. The traditional fixed playground equipment is there, but is of little interest to many of the children. A small stream has been dammed to form a fountain, then run under a wooden bridge, and it is ideal for splashing and water games; and a sandpit, five feet deep, is large enough for major excavations.

The lesson that the adventure playground offers to parents is that, as Keats said, "nothing is real until it is experienced." The child who has enjoyed cooking on a bonfire, playing out of his wheelchair on the ground, or splashing in water can take those experiences home with him. Adventure play is tough on the environment if a wheelchair is involved. Wheelchairs and braces catch doors and clothes. Grass is pulled up and clothes become filthy. But the paramount feature of the playground is the sense of adventure that it engenders in the children who use it.

Many children in wheelchairs are overcautious and timid. Their imagination needs stretching through experience, rather than through the vicarious thrills of the television. Hopefully the adventure playgrounds will encourage the family to see their child's potential for enjoyment in a different light, and will change the family's own attitude to recreation and vacation activities.

The Handicapped Adventure Playground movement has led to the development of specially landscaped and equipped playgrounds that offer a range of activities for disabled (and nondisabled) children and young people. They permit risk-taking in a range of indoor and outdoor activities under proper supervision and enable children who would otherwise have restricted access to adventure to learn new skills while having fun.

Even if it is impossible to replicate an adventure playground, many of the basic experiences of physical play for handicapped children can be applied in the home or school setting.

DESIGNING SPECIAL PLAY EQUIPMENT AND AIDS

Because their needs are so individual, many handicapped children need specially adapted play and other equipment. Since it is uneconomic for manufacturers to produce individual models, this will mean adaptation and modification. Parents are, not unnaturally, concerned about who can carry out these modifications or redesign a basic toy or piece of equipment. A new organization, consisting of therapists, engineers, teachers, and parents, was funded in the early 1970's to encourage cooperation in the construction and adaptation of aids, toys, and, educational material. Project Active* accepted that these aids to full participation in an effective educational program and play activities could never be mass-produced, and that the consumers and producers would therefore have to work together to identify unmet needs and devise methods of meeting

*Project Active is funded by the U.S. Office of Special Education. Information can be obtained from Thomas Vodola, 3213 Sharpe Rd., Wall, N.J. 07719 or Anthony Vodola, 3213 Danskin Rd., Wall Township, NJ 07719.

these. *Active* can offer itself as a referral agency to parents or professionals seeking a particular piece of equipment and publishes newsletters and holds regular workshops and meetings to discuss major issues.

Although parents feel nervous at the prospect of consulting specialist departments there is a variety of expertise which is relatively underused. Highly specialized and prototype equipment is very labor-intensive, and it is unlikely that it will be financially viable *unless* the free labor of a university, vocational, or technical design department is used. A number of technical schools and other college departments are now interested in designing for individual handicapped children and will sometimes organize "parent workshops" to explore designs and make prototypes for electronic toys, gadgets, and adaptations for disabled living.

LEISURE TIME AND HOBBIES

Gardening

The idea of gardening from a wheelchair may seem a contradiction. But gardening can be one of the major pleasures for a physically handicapped person, since it offers a unique opportunity for controlling one's own personal environment—even if that personal environment is a window box or a couple of tubs on a back terrace! The problems of the elderly in maintaining their ability to garden have produced a number of solutions for the difficulties experienced by younger handicapped people.

Raised beds can be made very cheaply, either by using garden stone or bricks to make raised troughs around the edge of a paved or concrete area suitable for wheelchair access, or by raising suitable containers on brick or other firm foundations: Old car tires piled on top of each other to a suitable height and painted or sprayed in white or a gay color make very good and cheap containers. If they are filled with earth and potting compost, they can support attractive groups of flowers. Baby baths or old sinks can also be used (the former being pierced to permit water to drain away). Gro-bags are available from most garden centers or shops. These long bags contain mineral and fertilizer-enriched compost and can be laid on any flat surface. The bag is pierced at regular intervals and the plants are set in. Because of the high nutrient value of the compost, vegetables such as tomatoes and potatoes, as well as flowers, can be grown with minimum attention and regular watering. A number of garden centers also sell *hydroponic* systems, in which plants and vegetables can be grown in special containers. No soil is used, but a filter bed with water and additions of suitable liquid fertilizers. This method of cultivation is particularly suitable for flats or for indoor gardening, when mess needs to be kept to a minimum. Climbing plants such as clematis, Russian vine, and roses can be trained up walls, so that their maintenance (once established) can be carried out from a wheelchair. If there is no external access, window boxes or house plants (including perhaps the miniature Japanese trees, the Bonsai) can provide interest.

Bird Watching

Children who cannot leave their house or yard frequently can get great enjoyment from bird watching. Simple bird feeders or bird houses, with a good stock of nuts, pieces of fat, coconut shells, bread, or bird seed, will ensure regular callers throughout the year. Net bags of nuts can be purchased from most pet shops and secured to a window by a suction cup. There are a number of attractive illustrated books on birds in children's book shops.

Fur and Feather—Pets for the Wheelchair Child

Although many people may feel that the suggestion of pets for disabled children is unrealistic, pets can play an important role for all children. For the child in a wheelchair, in particular, they mean responsibility for something else that is alive. Handicapped children become accustomed from a very early age to constant handling. Their bodies are examined, prodded, dressed, and undressed, and they are constantly moved and bundled around. In a sense they become objects and can avoid real decisions or responsibilities because of the need to wait for the next bit of help. "Thinking handicapped" is very easy if you do not have any responsibility. But pets—given that the right pet is chosen—can offer this feeling of reality and duty and encourage the child to realize the implications of any caring relationship.

If families have room in the house and a yard, they may be able to keep dogs and cats. But since these are fundamentally outdoor animals, the degree to which children in a wheelchair can take part in their physical care may be strictly limited. Fish are attractive, clean, and require minimal attention; but they also offer no personalized contact. So smaller animals, such as guinea pigs and hamsters, may prove the most satisfying pets. They are tame, good humored, sit comfortably in the lap, and can easily be housed in cages which can be placed at waist height for easy attention.

Another advantage of a pet is the attraction which it will offer to other children in the neighborhood. Animals invariably serve as a focus for discussion and activity, and offer a very normal family occupation. Most of the small animals are relatively cheap to keep. Families living in city areas where roadside grass cannot be gathered for food and bedding will have to purchase food and bedding straw at pet shops. But the smaller rodents live very happily on a diet mainly composed of vegetable scraps and offer little problem during vacation times. A hand-sized pet can be particularly useful if a child is immobilized for any period of time recovering from orthopedic surgery or general illness, since it can be handled and cared for without great physical effort.

Birds are also popular and practical. They are ornamental and require very little care. With attention, they can become tame and offer interest and color for a child. Cages can often be purchased second-hand and the general feeding costs are minimal.

SWIMMING

Water is the one really mobile environment for all handicapped people. Limbs which are rigid on land can float and move with the support of water, and many children will enjoy their first sensation of free movement in the swimming pool. Like all children, young disabled children should start to play in water from the earliest age. Many hospitals have hydrotherapy pools, where the water is used as an extra tool for the physical therapists. Most special schools also have access to pools and arrange weekly trips for regular swimming sessions. Special advice on teaching the young handicapped child to swim is offered. Very small children can easily be lifted in and out of the water wearing conventional swimming aids. However, it should be remembered that some children will have difficulty in turning themselves (if, for example, they slip over in a rubber ring), and care should be taken that buoyancy aids are safe. The absence of muscular control in the legs is not important in swimming; many strong swimmers have had no legs at all. But confidence and common sense are important, particularly when the child is bold enough to swim in lakes or the sea where currents and waves may cause extra hazards. It is also important to remember that children whose swimming experience is limited to calm, heated pools may not manage so well in turbulent or cold water. This is particularly true in the case of cerebral palsy or some type of paraplegia, where cold may cause an increase in spasm which makes swimming almost impossible. Hypothermia is also a risk, since paraplegics will not notice the side effects of poor circulation and cold water on their paralyzed limbs. This can occur even in indoor pools, particularly if the unheated water is at a low temperature on a cool summer's day.

An increasing number of handicapped children are enjoying other water sports, for which swimming is a prerequisite requirement. Unfortunately, sailing and rowing boats capsize, and care should be taken that children who are competent swimmers in an indoor pool really do have survival skills when accidentally immersed. Many spina bifida children, when sailing, will prefer to wear braces. Children with limb deficiencies may prefer to keep their prostheses (artificial limbs) on to maintain their mobility. Certain kinds of appliances are extremely heavy, and when combined with waterlogged clothing, will make swimming difficult if not impossible. It has been recommended that safety can be ensured by adding buoyancy devices to the braces or limbs to ensure that they will float on top of the water. If this is done without careful thought, the result may be that the legs tip up and float on the water and the child is pushed under, or held in a face downwards position in the water. Not all life jackets will function properly if other buoyancy aids are used, and it may be worth experimenting in an enclosed pool before venturing out in a lake or the ocean. It is, in fact, basic common sense to try out *all* children's lifejackets and buoyancy aids in a safe environment before letting them be used in the ocean. It should also be remembered that swimming as a means to survival in case of accident may involve learning techniques additional to conventional swimming skills. This is particularly important for handicapped people who may have great difficulty in climbing aboard a capsized boat, or (if they get into difficulties) in swimming against an undercurrent or tide. However, the best protection is proper instruction and supervision. Also, sailing and rowing should be learned from competent and experienced instructors.

Some children who become good swimmers will wish to proceed to the most sophisticated water sports. Diving is now practiced by a number of paraplegics, who find that their restrictions on land do not affect their movement in the water. Snorkeling is universally popular with small children, who enjoy wearing a mask and breathing tube or snorkel to make it possible to swim on the surface without lifting the head to breathe. This may be a special advantage for some children whose neck control is poor, or have difficulty in turning onto their side. However, snorkels have potential dangers for all users. If the mask does not seal properly over the eyes and mouth, water will leak in and upset breathing and vision. Face plates should be of unbreakable or shatterproof material, and be large enough to give unrestricted vision. Snorkels over 18 in. long are clumsy and may cause problems. Flippers can be used even on paralyzed limbs to give some residual movement, but care should be taken to protect legs and arms from scrapes on the bottom or sides of the pool. Any new equipment should at first be tried out under *close* supervision, and the child should understand the point of the design and the need to attach the snorkel and mask correctly. Disabled children are no more likely to injure themselves doing more adventurous swimming than their able-bodied friends, but they are at risk if they are required to move suddenly and quickly because apparatus has gone wrong. This is particularly true when swimming in the sea, where there may be a time gap between supervisors realizing a child is in difficulty and going to his rescue.

Some parents are worried about finding a "safe" pool for their children. Most swimming pools now have special sessions (and often free instruction) for handicapped swimmers. Some children who are very self-conscious may prefer these sessions. But others will quite naturally want to swim wherever *they* prefer. If the pool's management is anxious about safety risks, they may try and insist on special sessions only. If this happens, parents and the manager of the pool should discuss the issue and find a solution. Some pools are frightened of potential claim for damages if an accident occurs, but most are now willing and enthusiastic to help disabled people swim.

Sailing courses are now being run in a number of centers. Obviously a child in a wheelchair will wish to get out of his wheelchair and experience a normal sporting experience with his friends. However, early courses have shown not only success, but also possible problem areas. Paraplegics and spina bifida children have to take care to avoid accidental injury to their paralyzed limbs. They may need extra protective padding in the boat and perhaps wear wet suits which protect against cold and poor circulation as well as scratches and bruises.

Most disabled people will find a larger rather than a smaller boat comfortable, and some may find it impossible to balance on the seats. Suitable waterproof inflatable or foam cushions on the floor of the boat may therefore be needed. Care should be taken to avoid falls when balance is poor, and great care should be taken getting in and out of the boat. But, if basic safety precautions are observed, messing about in boats is just as possible and enjoyable for the disabled child as it is for all children.

VACATIONS

Everybody needs a vacation—children and parents, and sometimes each quite separately from the other. It can be a very hard decision for parents to agree to let their child go for a vacation without them—they feel torn between the desire to care for their child and their own (often guilty) need for a break. In fact, children often benefit more than the parents. A disabled child may live in an apartment in an urban area. If his parents do not have a car, outings will be strictly limited to the immediate neighborhood. There will be little chance of making friends, playing sports, swimming, and trying new activities. A handicapped child may *need* the independence of an unaccompanied vacation, especially as he reaches adolescence.

A number of voluntary organizations organize vacations which offer a real opportunity for enjoyment combined with a high standard of care. The choice of a suitable hotel or boarding house may mean that a child can go away with grandparents or friends exactly as he could if there were no wheelchair barrier. Many vacation camps can make special provision for wheelchairs and offer a range of activities. The voluntary organizations themselves frequently own vacation cabins with suitable modifications, which offer a very cheap vacation for a whole family or a group of friends.

Although parents often feel embarrassed at the suggestion that their child should have a vacation away from home, it may be useful for both the child (who may be able to try sports and activities in a special center which are unavailable at home) and for the parents and other members of the family. All the different members of an able-bodied family have their own interests, and it is fair that opportunity should be fairly divided. If a family likes mountain walking, scuba diving, or simply having individual vacations, their choice is not necessarily selfish for being met. Many parents of able-bodied chidren feel that they sometimes want to get away and have an "adult" vacation. If the handicapped child is particularly demeaning or severely handicapped, the need to have a complete rest may be very real. Tired parents are rarely good parents, and *all* members of the family may benefit from having a change of environment. There is no reason, in many cases, why the handicapped child should not have two vacations (one with the family, one without) if this seems a useful choice. An increasing number of special schools and clubs now organize summer camps and vacation plans; provided that the child is willing, it may stretch his horizons to get away and (perhaps for the first time) to have to fend more for himself.

If older children want a more structured vacation, there are a number of special centers which offer sporting and craft activities. Participants can join in a range of sports, including sailing, riding, canoeing, and caving. Clearly the degree of disability will dictate the amount of participation, but many disabled children are capable of managing rough ground and very basic vacation accommodations —particularly if they are capable of walking for short distances with aids.

Some centers offer opportunities for field studies, although the degree of activity again depends upon the mobility of the child. However, the use of electric wheelchairs has considerably extended the range of many children, and their potential enjoyment is considerable.

Wheelchair children because of their physical limitations, are often good observers, and an interest in natural history, geology, geography, and ancillary subjects can be lifelong—even if the most rural terrain in the neighborhood is the local park.

Camping and wheelchairs may seem incompatible, but an increasing number of projects are including children in wheelchairs in tent vacations. Camp and pack vacations are run by many Girl Scout troops. If extension group members (handicapped girls) are included, extra helpers and a nurse are provided.

HORSEBACK RIDING FOR THE DISABLED

Horseback riding has proved to be one of the most successful and enjoyable sports for physically and mentally handicapped children. Riding offers a unique opportunity to enjoy an outside sport, with the pleasure of a relationship with an animal. Most children love

236

horses, and find all aspects of their care—from cleaning out the stable to brushing and grooming—exciting. Riding offers a new environment and usually presents very few problems. Many riding schools are interested in helping, and provided that the rider can be mounted onto the horse without difficulty, no special facilities are needed. Needless to say, children should always wear hard hats and, initially, it is best to have two helpers per child (one to lead the horse and one to ensure that the child does not slip and fall). Special saddles can be purchased which have high pommels and cantles (rather like the American cowboy saddle). Some have back rests for children with weak spines.

Helpers do not all have to be "horsey" people, although knowledge of horses, their equipment, and basic riding techniques is useful. The importance of the exercise is to give other physically handicapped children the experience described by one handicapped girl— "Freedom is what riding means to me. To be able to move about where I want to without having to ask someone to give me a push." Many children feel free on horseback in a way that they feel nowhere else except in the water. There is clearly a demand, and a great satisfaction in sitting on a warm horse's back and enjoying the pattern of movement. Not everybody will be able to emulate the success of Lis Hartel, who won a silver medal for Dressage in the 1952 Olympic Games, although very severely disabled by poliomyelitis. Nevertheless a number of wheelchair children have managed pony treks and unaccompanied riding—and innumerable others have improved their balance and coordination by sharing a sport with the able-bodied.

WHEELCHAIR SPORTS

The Special Olympics are now a regular fixture in the sporting calendar. Although some people feel strongly that integrated sports or activities are all-important, it is obvious tht some activities must be separate to be equal. However, wheelchair sports can include archery, volleyball, swimming, javelin throwing, and horseback riding. A number of international competitions are staged every year, and many disabled people can, of course, compete equally at sports like table tennis or archery. Some children play cricket or football from a wheelchair or with crutches. But whether sport is competitive or just fun, it is useful to strengthen muscles and give the child a chance to meet other people. Many schools have sports clubs, and some kind of training in a segregated setting may be helpful before going on to the local youth club's table tennis tournament or swimming relay race.

The Special Olympics was created and developed by the Joseph P. Kennedy, Jr., Foundation in 1968 to give mentally retarded children from the age of eight and up the opportunity to compete in a sports program. The mission of Special Olympics is to provide year-round sports training and athletic competition in a variety of well-coached Olympic-type sports for all mentally retarded children and adults, giving them continuing opportunities to develop physical fitness, express courage, experience joy, and participate in a sharing of gifts, skills, and friendship with their families, other Special Olympians, and the community (*Official Special Olympics Sports Rules*, 1980).

Today Special Olympics has spread to every state in the United States, to every province of Canada, to France, and to Puerto Rico. Many universities and community organizations have begun to participate and support the Special Olympics program in their own state. To find out more about Special Olympics or the name of your state Special Olympics director contact. Mrs. Eunice Kennedy Shriver, President, Special Olympics, Inc., Joseph P. Kennedy, Jr., Foundation, 1701 K Street, NW, Washington, D. C. 20006.

SCOUTS

Scouting is available throughout the country, and offers excellent opportunities for handicapped children to make friends and participate in "normal" activities. Scout headquarters have a headquarter commissioner and assistant commissioner for extension activities. Camping and general outdoor scouting activities are also open to the handicapped, although it may be necessary for a wheelchair child in a wheelchair to attend a county rather than a district camp if a good deal of special help is needed. The emphasis is, however, on integration, and handicapped children are never excluded from any activity unnecessarily.

The Girl Scouts also welcomes handicapped girls in local troops. Special extension units are also organized, mainly based in special schools and hospitals. Girls are welcome on camps and outings and normal scouting activities, and those who live too far away to attend a local unit can be scouts by mail.

Many local youth clubs accept handicapped members as they accept any other interested member of the community. If transportation is a problem, social services or local voluntary organizations can sometimes provide volunteers to help. It is always worth contacting a local branch of a voluntary organization to see if there are local groups.

Joining clubs may seem very hard to work to parents if they have to take their child some distance. It may, in some cases, be hard to persuade the handicapped child to get out and make the effort to meet new people and try new activities. But it is very unwise to let a child stay at home unnecessarily, relying solely on his family for fun and entertainment. The ability to make friends is based largely upon opportunity and practice: Far too many handicapped children appear gauche and dependent precisely because they *are* dependent and have little chance to think and act independently.

Clubs may pose particular problems in rural areas, where transportation is a difficulty and rides difficult to obtain, but in these cases it is worth persevering and asking through a local church, club, or other charitable organization, if anybody can provide a ride. Since public transport is getting scarcer in many parts of the country, more people are having to rely on cars and there is possibly more opportunity of finding cars going in the right direction.

MUSIC AND MUSIC CLUBS

The majority of handicapped children can learn instruments and play in orchestras or groups exactly like their able-bodied counterparts. Music is a satisfying art—either for solo pleasure or for social activities—and it is worth making an effort to ensure that children have the opportunity to learn an instrument. Many local music groups and clubs are willing to accept disabled children, and notices can usually be found in libraries and local papers.

Most libraries have record sections, and listening to music can also be a pleasurable activity. Access to live concerts can be more of a problem. Many musical events outside large cities take place in old premises where access to the auditorium, restaurant, and restrooms may be extremely inconvenient. Many local handicap groups have done local surveys of physical access to public buildings, shops, restrooms, and so forth, but if no such survey is available, advance inspection may be necessary. If necessary, and if there are two helpers, many wheelchair children can be "walked" for limited distances or carried (walking with canes, crutches, or a walker is often as difficult as managing a wheelchair, if there are many steps and

239

corners to negotiate and if the lighting is bad). Many concert halls and theaters have service elevators, and these can often be utilized if the manager is contacted first.

Music therapy is often used to help physically handicapped children both with movement and emotional problems. Music therapy may be available through a local school or hospital, or parents can find their own therapist. Music therapists, contrary to many people's notions, are professionally trained both in music and in the therapeutic application of their musical knowledge, and offer as professional a service as speech therapists or occupational therapists. Paul Nordoff, a composer who died in 1976, extended the principle of music therapy to very severely physically and mentally handicapped children through the Nordoff Music Therapy Centre. Parents who feel that they cannot afford personal therapists, but are interested in music as a means of communication, can sometimes employ a therapist for a group and make the therapy a regular sessional activity.

Another music-based activity is dancing. *Wheelchair dancing* developed by chance out of movements to music designed to encourage more effective management of wheelchairs. Wheelchair dancing has become extremely popular, with elaborate dance routines and a number of public performances. There is no reason why wheelchair dancers should not dance with able-bodied partners, and dancing and discos are regular parts of many club activities.

Many clubs organize social activities, and parents might remember that a shy teenager, who is reluctant to brave the social world in a wheelchair, might enjoy having a party himself or herself. It is often easier to be host than guest, and many voluntary organizations have recognized the need for the normal social activities and parties that all teenagers enjoy. Clubs are not merely means of developing new interests. They are ways of making individual relationships, and it is this ongoing development of friendship and chosen activities which handicapped adolescents will often miss out on, unless their parents are very willing to help and encourage. It may be very hard to know, when you go out, that you have to come home with father or travel in a minibus at a prearranged time. It is equally hard not to be able to disappear in a snack bar without forethought and planning. But the end product of club going should be more young people *at home*, and, despite the noise, dirty coffee cups, and late nights, parents will want to think about these needs.

PRIVATE PLEASURES

Everybody needs a hobby which they can do on their own, and wheelchair children are no exception. Collecting stamps is a hobby which can be expensive and complicated, or cheap and simple. Many towns have local groups and clubs. Jigsaw puzzles, too, are amusing and relaxing for many people.

Chess is a popular game—or sport—for many adolescents, who can play in local and specialist chess clubs and events. A wide range of paperback guides to the game are available, and self-instruction is not difficult. Some children may find small chess figures difficult to manipulate, but the wide range of commercially produced sets should make it possible to find a suitable set.

Printing is often popular, and has the advantage of being a potentially profitable hobby since small printing sets can be purchased quite cheaply and can be used to print school concert programs, tickets, and letter headings. Many local authorities offer evening classes in printing, and a number of schools, workshops, and day centers have small machines. These machines can be modified to be operated by foot as well as by hand.

Reading is usually a pleasure for all age groups, and few areas of the country are inaccessible to good children's libraries. A number of special books are now available on children in wheelchairs, including Camilla Jessel's photographic adventure story, *Mark's Wheelchair Adventures* (Methuen) and Elizabeth Fanshawe's *Rachel*, a picture story for younger children (published by Bodley Head). Children about to go into the hospital may enjoy books on hospital themes. These following books are about children with physical handicaps:

Killilea Marie. *Wren.* Dell Publishing Co.

Little, Jean. *Mine for Keeps.* Little, Brown & Co.

Fassler, Joan. *Howie Helps Himself.* Albert Whitman & Co.

Savitz, Harriet May. *Fly, Wheels, Fly.* John Day.

Wolf, Bernard. *Don't Feel Sorry for Paul.* Lippincott; Harper & Row.

Patterson, Kathryn. *No Time for Fears.* Johnson Publishing.

Neufield, John. *Touching.* S. G. Phillips.

Savitz, Harriet May. *On the Move.* Avon.

If a child has sight problems, most libraries can lend large-print books. Occasionally handicapped children may be immobilized on their backs and unable to read because they cannot raise their head sufficiently. Prismatic spectacles can be purchased through opticians (either in plain glass or made up to an individual prescription). These glasses work like a periscope so that the person concerned can see things at right angles to their direct line of vision. Tables can be purchased which operate on a cantilever system so that the table can be tipped and a book placed at a convenient angle. Pages, if hand control is poor, may be easier to turn if rubber thimbles are worn (available from stationers for counting money and sorting papers), or if a spoon handle or paper clip is used. Unicorn sticks on a headband can be obtained or manufactured at home if there is no hand control.

"Talking books" are usually thought of as being relevant to blind people only. They are useful for anybody whose sight or physical control of a book or journal is inadequate. Handicapped students requiring some visual representation of tables or diagrams may need a microfilm projector for filmed books and papers.

Parents and other members of the family can record material themselves, if they have the time available. Tapes can be used a number of times, and although taping a whole novel is time consuming, many children's stories, songs, or news items can be taped fairly quickly.

Arts and crafts can generally be practiced by the able-bodied and handicapped at home. Although fine finger control is required for embroidery and elaborate needlework, many children can learn to make simple clothes like wraparound skirts on a sewing machine. Electric sewing machines can be modified to work by hand rather than foot pressure, but some children will find the old hand sewing machines easier to manage. They can be purchased quite cheaply secondhand.

If it is not possible to find a special arts and craft teacher locally, many adult education courses now have Saturday or early evening sessions in particular crafts which a handicapped older child could attend. Some children will not wish to take a craft very seriously, but merely to use it as an occupation and recreation. Others may become very involved in collages, pottery, or wood carving, and will gain from professional teaching. Papier-maché, clay, and other modeling and craft products can be purchased through a number of large toy or art shops, or by mail order from special children's shops. Crafts encourage children to use their hands and develop fine finger control, and they have an attractive end product.

Children, needless to say, should have some say in what they do, and should have the opportunity to try and discard a range of activities. With increasing unemployment, and earlier retirement, leisure activities are assuming a new importance for everybody. Leisure counseling, in fact, is a new need and handicapped people in particular (who are likely to have to spend more time on their own than most people, and to have the greatest difficulty in obtaining work) need to develop a wide range of hobbies. These hobbies should be the children's, and parents should beware of jumping in and completing the pressed flower arrangment or the piece of crochet. Hobbies are for life, and nobody will need them more than a severely handicapped or chronically sick person whose outside activities are likely to remain severely restricted.

Appendix A

Organizations and Agencies Serving Children and Adults with Handicaps

Adapted Sports Association, Inc.
6832 Marlette
Marlette, Michigan 48453

Alexander Graham Bell Association for the Deaf
3417 Volta Place, N.W.
Washington, D.C. 20007

American Alliance for Health, Physical Education, Recreation, and Dance
1900 Association Drive
Reston, Virginia 22091

American Association on Mental Deficiency
5101 Wisconsin Avenue
Washington, D.C. 20016

American Athletic Association for the Deaf
3916 Lantern Drive
Silver Spring, Maryland 20902

American Blind Bowling Association
Bradford Woods
Martinsville, Indiana 46151

American Camping Association
Bradford Woods
Martinsville, Indiana 46151

American Coalition of Citizens with Disabilities
1346 Connecticut Ave., N.W. Suite 1124
Washington, D.C. 20036

American Council for the Blind
1211 Connecticut Avenue, N.W.
Washington, D.C. 20036

American Foundation for the Blind, Inc.
15 West 16th Street
New York, New York 10011

American Occupational Therapy Association
1383 Piccard Drive
Rockville, Maryland 20580

American Orthotic and Prosthetic Association
1440 N Street, N.W.
Washington, D.C. 20005

American Physical Therapy Association
1156 15th Street, N.W.
Washington, D.C. 20005

American Printing House for the Blind
P.O. Box 6085
Louisville, Kentucky 40206

American Speech and Hearing Association
10801 Rockville Pike
Rockville, Maryland 20852

American Wheelchair Bowling Association
6718 Pinehurst Drive
Evansville, Indiana 47711

American Wheelchair Pilots Association
P.O. Box 1181
Mesa, Arizona 85201

Amputee Sports Association
11705 Mercy Boulevard
Savannah, Georgia 31406

Association for Children with Learning Disabilities
4156 Library Road
Pittsburgh, Pennsylvania 15234

Association for Education of the Visually Handicapped
919 Walnut Street, Fourth Floor
Philadelphia, Pennsylvania 19107

Association of Foot and Mouth Painters
503 Brisband Building
Buffalo, New York 10403

Blind Outdoor Leisure Development
533 East Main Street
Aspen, Colorado 81611

Boy Scouts of America
Scouting for the Handicapped Division
U.S. Routes 1 and 30
North Brunswick, New Jersey 08902

Coalition on Sexuality and Disability
122 East 23rd Street
New York, New York 10010

Columbia Lighthouse for the Blind
421 P Street, N.W.
Washington, D.C. 20005

Council for Exceptional Children
1920 Association Drive
Reston, Virginia 22091

Council of Education of the Deaf
c/o Gallaudet College
Seventh Street and Florida Avenue
Washington, D.C. 20002

Cystic Fibrosis Foundation
6000 Executive Boulevard Suite 309
Rockville, Maryland 20852

Dental Guidance Council for Cerebral Palsy
122 East 23rd Street
New York, New York 10010

Disabled Sportsmen of America
P.O. Box 26
Vinton, Virginia 24179

Down's Syndrome Congress
1640 West Roosevelt Road
Chicago, Illinois 60608

Dysautonomia Foundation, Inc.
370 Lexington Avenue
New York, New York 10017

Ephphatha Services for the Deaf and Blind
421 South 4th Street
P.O. Box 15167
Minneapolis, Minnesota 55415

Epilepsy Foundation of America
1828 L Street, Suite 405
Washington, D.C. 20036

Federation of the Handicapped
211 West 14th Street
New York, New York 10011

Foundation for Children with Learning Disabilities
99 Park Avenue, 2nd Floor
New York, New York 10011

Friedreich's Ataxia Group in America
P.O. Box 11116
Oakland, California 94611

Girl Scouts of the USA
Scouting for Handicapped Girls
830 Third Avenue
New York, New York 10022

Handicapped Boaters Association
P.O. Box 1134
Ansonia Station, New York 10023

International Association of Parents of the Deaf
814 Thayer Avenue
Silver Spring, Maryland 20910

International Committee of the Silent Sports
Gallaudet College
Florida Avenue and 7th St. N.E.
Washington, D.C. 20002

International Handicappers' Net
(Ham Radio Operators)
717 Anderson Way
San Gabriel, California 91776

International Spinal Cord Research Foundation
4100 Spring Valley Road, Suite 104 LB3
Dallas, Texas 75234

International Wheelchair Road Racers Club(IWRRC)
12710 N. 30th Street, #147
Tampa, Florida 33612

John Tracy Clinic
(Deafness/Hearing Impairments, Deaf-Blind)
806 West Adams Boulevard
Los Angeles, California 90007

Juvenile Diabetes Association
23 East 26th Street
New York, New York 10010

Leukemia Society of America
800 Second Avenue
New York, New York 10017

Louis Braille Foundation for Blind Musicians
215 Park Avenue South
New York, New York 10003

Mainstream Information Center
1200 15th Street, N.W.
Washington, D.C. 20005

Mobility International USA
P.O. Box 3551
Eugene, Oregon 97403

Muscular Dystrophy Association, Inc.
810 Seventh Avenue
New York, New York 10019

National Amputation Foundation
12-45 150th Street
Whitestone, New York 11357

National Arts and the Handicapped Information Service
National Endowment for the Arts
2401 E Street, N.W.
Washington, D.C. 20506

National Association for Down's Syndrome
Box 63
Oak Park, Illinois 60303

National Association of the Deaf
814 Thayer Avenue
Silver Spring, Maryland 20910

National Association for Retarded Citizens
2501 Avenue J
P.O. Box 6109
Arlington, Texas 76011

National Association for the Visually Handicapped
305 East 24th Street, Room 17-C
New York, New York 10010

National Association for Sports for Cerebral Palsy
P.O. Box 3847 Amity Station
New Haven, Connecticut 06511

National Association of Private Residential Facilities
for the Mentally Retarded
6269 Leesburg Pike
Falls Church, Virginia 22204

National Association of Private Schools for Exceptional Children
P.O. Box 34293
West Bethesda, Maryland 20817

National Association of the Deaf-Blind
2703 Forest Oak Circle
Norman, Oklahoma 73071

National Association of the Physically Handicapped
76 Elm Street
London, Ohio 43140

National Ataxia Foundation
600 Twelve Oaks Center
15500 Wayzata Boulevard
Wayzata, Minnesota 55391

National Center for the Barrier-Free Environment
1140 Connecticut Avenue, Suite 1006
Washington, D.C. 20036

National Center for Law and the Handicapped
University of Notre Dame
P.O. Box 477
Notre Dame, Indiana 46556

National Committee on Arts for the Handicapped
1825 Connecticut Avenue, N.W.
Suite 418
Washington, D.C. 20009

National Congress of Organizations of the Physically Handicapped, Inc.
1627 Deborah Avenue
Rockford, Illinois 61103

National Easter Seal Society for Crippled Children and Adults
2023 Ogden Avenue
Chicago, Illinois 60612

National Federation of the Blind
1346 Connecticut Avenue, N.W.
Suite 212, Dupont Circle Building
Washington, D.C. 20036

National Foundation for Wheelchair Tennis
3055 Birch Street
Newport Beach, California 92660

National Foundation for Ileitis and Colitis
295 Madison Avenue
New York, New York 10017

National Foundation/March of Dimes
1275 Mamaroneck Avenue
White Plains, New York 10605

National Foundation of Dentistry for the Handicapped
1726 Champa, Suite 422
Denver, Colorado 80202

National Genetics Foundation
555 West 57th Street, Room 1240
New York, New York 10019

National Handicapped Sports and Recreation Association
Capitol Hill Station
P.O. Box 18664
Denver, Colorado 80218

National Hearing Aid Society
20361 Middlebelt Road
Livona, Michigan 48152

National Hemophilia Foundation
19 West 34th Street, Room 1204
New York, New York 10001

National Library Services for the Blind and Physically Handicapped
Library of Congress
1291 Taylor Street, N.W.
Washington, D.C. 20542

National Multiple Sclerosis Society
205 East 42nd Street
New York, New York 10017

National Neurofibromatosis Foundation
3401 Woodridge Court
Mitchellville, Maryland 20716

National Paraplegia Foundation
333 North Michigan Avenue
Chicago, Illinois 60601

National Retinitis Pigmentosa Foundation
Rolling Park Building
8311 Mindale Circle
Baltimore, Maryland 21207

National Society for Autistic Children
1234 Massachusetts Avenue, N.W.
Suite 1017
Washington, D.C. 20005

National Spinal Injury Foundation
369 Elliot Street
Newton Upper Falls, Massachusetts 02164

National Tay-Sachs and Allied Diseases Association
122 East 42nd Street
New York, New York 10068

National Tuberous Sclerosis Association
P.O. Box 159
Laguna Beach, California 92651

National Wheelchair Athletic Association
40-24 62nd Street
Woodside, New York 11377

National Wheelchair Basketball Association
110 Seaton Building
University of Kentucky
Lexington, Kentucky 40506

National Wheelchair Marathon
380 Diamond Hill Road
Warwick, Rhode Island 02886

National Wheelchair Motorcycle Association
101 Torrey Street
Brockton, Massachusetts 03401

National Wheelchair Softball Association
P.O. Box 737
Sioux Falls, South Dakota 57101

North American Riding for the Handicapped Association, Inc.
P.O. Box 100
Ashburn, Virginia 22011

Orton Society (dyslexia)
8415 Bellona Lane
Towson, Maryland 21204

Performing Arts Theater for the Handicapped
5410 Wilshire Boulevard, Suite 510
Los Angeles, California 90036

Rehabilitation International USA
20 West 40th Street
New York, New York 10018

Society for the Rehabilitation of the Facially Disfigured
560 First Avenue
New York, New York 10016

Special Citizens Futures Unlimited (Autistic Adults)
823 United Nations Plaza
New York, New York 10017

Special Olympics, Inc.
Kennedy Foundation
1701 K Street, N.W., Suite 215
Washington, D.C. 20006

Spina Bifida Association of America
343 South Dearborn Street, Room 317
Chicago, Illinois 60604

Task Force on Life Safety and the Handicapped
P.O. Box 19044
Washington, D.C. 20036

Theater for the Deaf
University of Montana
Missoula, Montana 59801

Travel Information Center
Moss Rehabilitation Hospital
12th St. and Tabor Road
Philadelphia, Pennsylvania 19141

Tuberous Sclerosis Association of America
P.O. Box 44
Rockland, Massachusetts 02320

United Cerebral Palsy Association, Inc.
66 East 34th Street
New York, New York 10016

United Ostomy Association
2001 West Beverly Boulevard
Los Angeles, California 90057

United States Amputee Association
Route 2, County Line
Fairview, Tennessee 37062

United States Association for Blind Athletes
55 West California Avenue
Beach Haven Park, New Jersey 08008

United States Deaf Skiers Association
159 Davis Avenue
Hackensack, New Jersey 07601

Western Law Center for the Handicapped
849 South Broadway, Suite M-22
Los Angeles, California 90014

Appendix B

Manufacturers of Aids and Appliances Mentioned in the Text

Alvema Rehab (see Ortho-Kinetics, Inc.)

Amigo Sales, Inc.
6693 Dixie Highway
Bridgeport, Michigan 48722

BEC (Biddle Engineering Co. Ltd.)
103 Stourbridge Road
Halesowen, W. Midlands, England

Be OK!
Fred Sammons, Inc.
Box 32
Brookfield, Illinois 60513

Braune of Stroud (BATRIC)
Griffin Mill, Thrupp, Stroud
Gloucestershire GL5 2AZ, England

Childcraft
20 Kilmer Road
Edison, New Jersey 08818

Comfy Products
Comfort House
Marshall Avenue
Bridlington, Yorkshire, England

Desemo Inc.
P.O. Box 22309
Savannah, Georgia 31403

Everest & Jennings Preston
J. A. Preston Corp.
60 Page Road
Clifton, New Jersey 07102

Ted Hoyer & Co. Ltd.
2222 Minnesota Street
Oshkosh, Wisconsin 54901

Invacare
1200 Taylor Street
Elyria, Ohio 44035

Invacare
741 West 17th Street
Long Beach, California 90813

MECALIFT
Mecanaids Ltd.
St. Catherine Street
Gloucester, England

Modular Medical Corp.
177 East 87th Street
New York, New York 10028

L. Mulholland Corp.
215 North 12th Street
Santa Paula, California 93060

J. Nesbit-Evans & Co. Ltd.
Wednesbury, Staffs WS10 7BC, England

Nolan Tub & Pool Lifts
J. E. Nolan and Co., Inc.
Box 43201
Louisville, Kentucky 40243

Ortho-Kinetics, Inc.
P.O. Box 2000
Waukesha, Wisconsin 53187

J. A. Preston Corp.
60 Page Road
Clifton, New Jersey 07012

Schaper Playmobil
Constructive Playthings
2008 West 103rd Terrace
Leawood, Kansas 66206

Simplantex Products
Willowfield House
Eastbourne, Sussex, England

Sunflower Bathing Aids
Handcraft
Nottingham Handcraft Company
Melton Road
West Bridgford, Nottingham NG2 6HD, England

Suzy
Spastics Society
16 Fitzroy Square
London W. 1., England

Index